Tove Nilsson is a chef, food writer and sommelier. She is regularly commissioned for Sweden's leading food magazines and news programmes. Tove is often heard on the radio where she shares recipes and discusses the latest trends in the food world.

POP Bubble & FIZZ

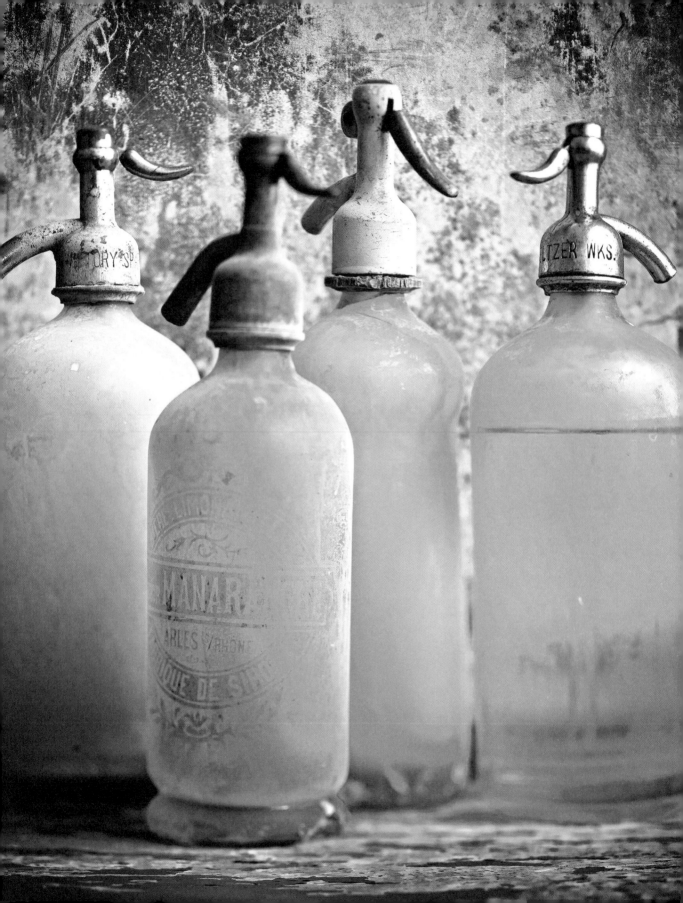

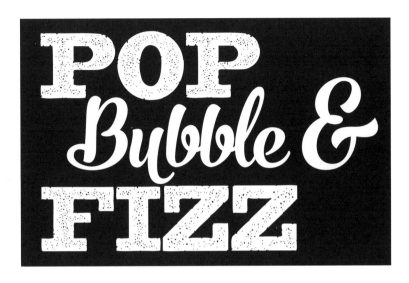

POP Bubble & FIZZ

RECIPES FOR HOMEMADE DRINKS & SNACKS

TOVE NILSSON

PHOTOGRAPHY BY WOLFGANG KLEINSCHMIDT

PAVILION

First published in the United Kingdom in 2015 by
Pavilion
1 Gower Street
London
WC1E 6HD

Copyright © 2014 Tove Nilsson
Natur & Kultur, Stockholm

ISBN 978-1-910496-26-8

A CIP catalogue record for this book is available from the British Library.

10 9 8 7 6 5 4 3 2 1

Reproduction by Mission Productions Ltd, Hong Kong
Printed by Craft Print Ltd, Singapore

This book can be ordered direct from the publisher at
www.pavilionbooks.com

Photography by Wolfgang Kleinschmidt
Designed by Katy Kimbell

This ... Made Up een for her
wo...

First published in 2014 by Natur & Kultur,
Stockholm ... Natur & Kultur

www.nok.se
info@nok.se

Publisher's note:
Always read the instructions carefully when using glass bottles and containers.

CONTENTS

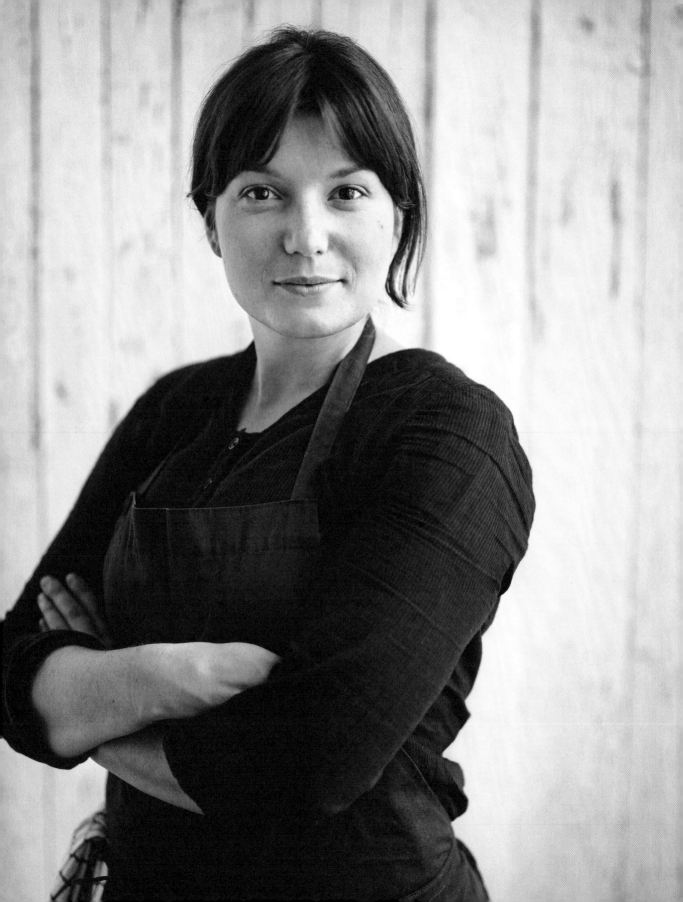

INTRODUCTION

I like ice-cold drinks and I'm particular when it comes to how cold they are. I stock up the freezer with ice and feel a bit down if I have to drink soda or lemonade without ice. Besides, if it's a soda, you don't get that same tickling feeling from the carbonic acid if the drink is lukewarm. Because that's the sensation I'm after – that prickly cold mouthful that gets the flavours going and quenches the thirst.

After working as a chef and a food writer for many years I trained as sommelier to learn more about combining food and drink. I soon realised that it's actually not only wine, decent beer and spirits that can match with the food, but also beverages flavoured with fruit, herbs and spices.

I'm on a constant hunt for exciting liquid flavours and experiences: the acidity in a perfectly balanced lemonade, the fresh taste of a melon and lime soda or the bitterness in a grapefruit-fermented soda.

My earliest memories of fizzy drinks go back to my childhood when I was allowed to go down into the larder in the basement and pick a bottle of pop from the red plastic crate. It stood on the shelf next to homemade cordial and marmalade.

I also remember the feeling of luxury when standing in the food store choosing which 24 fizzy pops we should fill the compartments with. My favourites were Swedish classics such as sugar soda, or raspberry or other fruit sodas.

My taste for fizzy drinks has changed over the years. Today I get more excited by drinks that have a lovely dry character with a good balance between acidity and sweetness. Once you've tried homemade soda it's difficult even to consider the sugar-infested fizzy pop you often get at the supermarket. The naturally fermented soda is a particular favourite. Through lacto-fermentation, the finished drink gets a deep flavour that's almost irresistible.

My hunt for drinks has taken me all over the world. In Mexico I gulped down buckets of cooling agua de sandía while crunching on freshly fried tortilla chips with guacamole sitting by tables covered with salsa-sticky wax cloths. I munched the occasional coriander-stuffed taco with a glass of agua de flor de Jamaica on the beach and, after dinners of spicy enchiladas, I sipped on a sickly sweet but oh-so-cooling horchata, made from rice and with a taste of cinnamon and vanilla, almost like a milkshake.

In the Amazon jungle I almost missed the flight back to Lima when I just had to try a glass of juice made from cashew apple that a local show owner had praised to high heaven. I still remember the taste, which was a bit nutty and creamy but still refreshing and cooling.

In Peru I drank the country's pride, Inca Kola, a poisonous-looking, bright yellow soda that tastes of bubblegum. It was frankly disgusting the first time I tried it, but after some time I couldn't be without it at the weekend. Once back home, the addiction slowly went away once the memories of the trip started to fade.

In England I've scoffed down piles of vinegar crisps while sipping iced tea and rose lemonade. And in Asia I've had sickly sweet bubble tea, a drink that comes with lots of slimy bubbles made from tapioca at the bottom. It doesn't sound very nice but, just like a Mexican horchata, can be compared to a milkshake or an iced tea with a lot of milk.

Nowadays I always have a batch of kombucha brewing in my kitchen after having tried it for the first time in the US – I was hooked after the first mouthful of the acidic fresh fermented tea.

I've drunk my way through a whole lot of what the world has to offer in refreshing alcohol-free beverages, but it's been through my travels to the US that I've realised that soda and fizzy drinks can be so much more than an artificially sweet, factory-produced drink: making them can be a real craft. In recent years I've noticed a trend towards using natural ingredients as a base and adding your own carbonated water, and brewing your own soda using natural fermentation. We are turning further away from the bottles of soda made with chemically produced corn syrup that were designed to travel long distances and instead using filtered tap water and Demerara sugar or molasses as a base.

From visiting small soda producers and soda fountains I've learned the basics of soda production using natural ingredients. And I've gathered all my notes here together with recipes for cooled lemonades and fruit beverages, and some tasty snacks to go with them. After a period of testing you can start swapping berries, fruit and spices to make your own flavour combinations. The important thing is to stick to the same ratio of yeast and soda to liquid to avoid over-fermenting and failed fermentation. Apart from that you'll just have to load up the freezer with ice and get started on the boiling, brewing, pressing and blending.

Good luck!
Tove

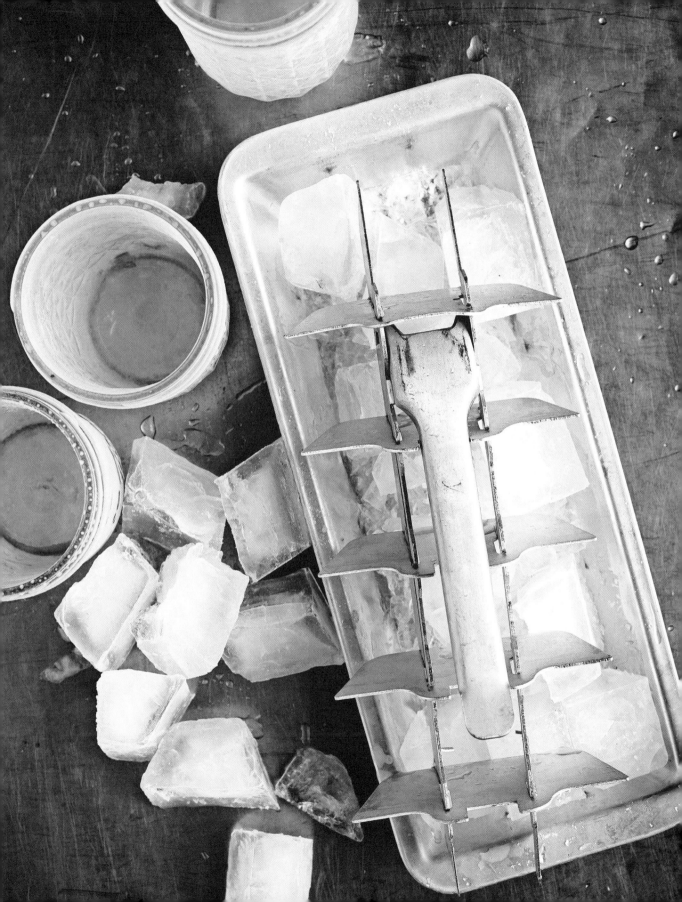

SODA
from
SCRATCH

It's easy to make your own soda. You don't need any advanced equipment and – in contrast to brewing beer, wine and cider – it's very quick to produce a tasty fizzy drink. If you just take it easy, follow the recipes and don't let yourself get upset if the first batch isn't completely successful, you'll be able to drink plenty of glasses of ice-cold soda.

I've created loads of recipes for different types of soda – some of which are quick and can be served up after 10 minutes and others that are a little more advanced and will need to go through a fermentation process in order to become bubbly and carbonated.

One tip is to read through the information on the next few pages carefully before you get started, as it will make it a lot easier to follow the recipes and then – after a little practice – start to create your own.

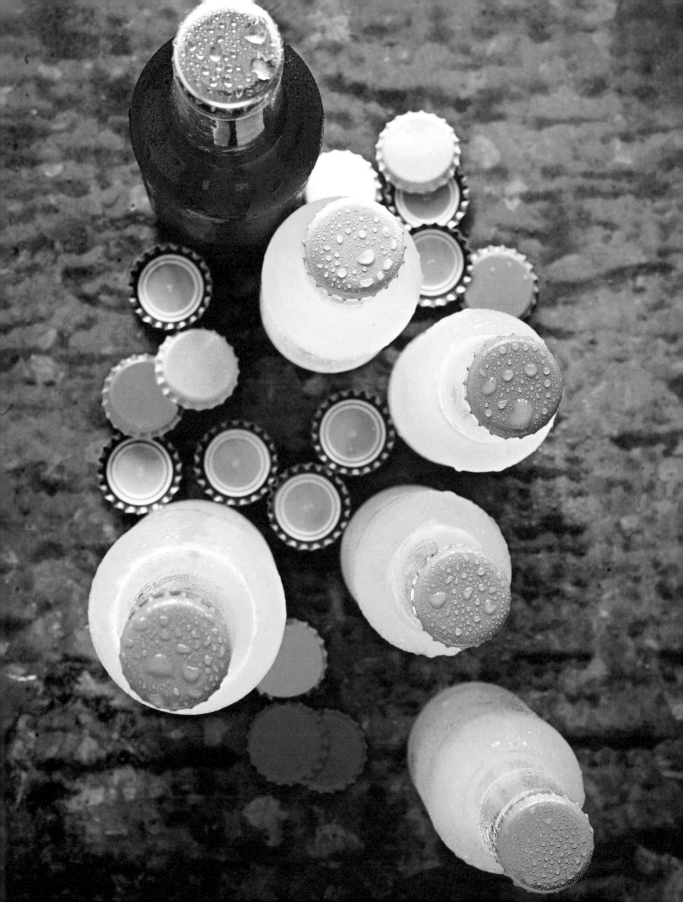

CARBONIC ACID

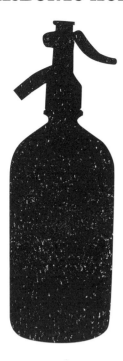

The important thing about soda is carbonic acid and there are several different ways to create these tasty bubbles. You can either mix together carbonated water with flavoured syrup, brew soda with yeast, or use natural fermentation.

The simplest technique is to use a soda maker or a classic soda siphon that can be found in department stores. With one of these and some soda syrup, you can mix your own drink, as you would with a cordial, and decide for yourself how concentrated a flavour you want. This is the classic technique and is pretty much what happens when you get a drink from a soda dispenser – a flavoured concentrate mixing with carbonated water. That's why coke can taste different depending on where you are, as any residual flavours in the water will flavour the drink.

Another technique is to brew the soda using yeast or through natural fermentation. When brewing with yeast I use liquid champagne or cider yeast. (The Edelmans and Wyeast brands give the least amount of residual flavour.) After many tests using normal baker's yeast and beer yeast, I decided that there isn't any alternative to the champagne yeast, since the soda simply didn't end up tasting nice.

A lot of people might think it sounds complicated to brew with yeast, but it's not. You mix together a tasty juice as a base – from fruit, spices or berries – then simply add a little yeast. The important thing is not to add too much or you could get an explosion in your kitchen!

The third technique, in which everything is made from scratch without any additives, is the one I like the best. Here you lacto-ferment the soda, just like when making sauerkraut, kimchi or other fermented vegetables. The end result is a bubbly soda with a fantastic flavour and character.

Another thing that's good about this technique is that it's possible to ferment the soda until it is almost completely dry. For this, you leave the soda in the glass jar to ferment for a little longer, while checking the flavours from time to time. The sugar is eaten by the soda culture and contributes to the tasty bubbles in the final drink.

You start by making a soda culture, almost like a sourdough. The soda culture is built from three ingredients: water, ginger and sugar. The culture needs to be fed every day and after about three to five days you have a bubbly liquid that can be mixed with fruit juice. After a few days of fermentation the fruit juice will transform into carbonated soda.

WATER

It doesn't actually matter what kind of water you use, the end result will be about the same. The difference lies in which type of minerals the water contains and its pH values, which of course will contribute to a slight variation in flavour and sensation. When the water is mixed with flavoured soda the difference becomes almost insignificant. Use whichever water you want for the recipes in this book.

SODA or FIZZY POP

Soda and fizzy pop are really the same thing. Soda is a more international word for fizzy pop and is the term used in the US. I think it sounds a bit nicer to say homemade ice-cold soda than fizzy pop or fizzy drink.

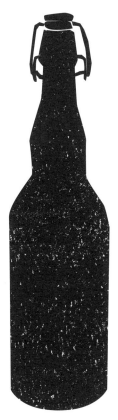

ALCOHOL

A by-product of fermentation is alcohol and there is always some alcohol in all types of fermented products. That goes for soda and elderflower champagne, but also for sauerkraut, sourdough bread and kimchi. You don't have to worry about high alcohol content, however, since the soda contains such a small amount of yeast and is brewed in such a short time that the alcohol content will never get higher than 1 percent. The soda can't ferment for long, as it would explode from the carbonic acid that fills up the bottle. The fermentation is stalled before all the sugar has been eaten by the yeast, which is why the soda never reaches a higher alcohol content.

It's quite natural that the finished soda tastes and smells a bit of yeast, but this doesn't mean it contains a lot of alcohol.

Soda made from soda syrup is not fermented and can be regarded as cordial that is mixed with carbonated water, therefore totally alcohol-free.

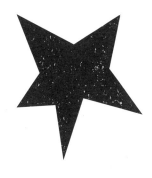

EXPLOSIONS *when* BREWING AT HOME

When brewing with yeast and soda culture, the live yeast bacteria are thriving in the liquid. The sugar and the fruit are eaten by the bacteria and the by-products are carbonic acid and alcohol. The more yeast and the longer time the soda ferments, the more carbonic acid and risk of an explosion.

When I developed the recipes for this book I tried out different amounts of yeast and soda culture to get the absolute best results. A few times I came to work in the mornings and was greeted by grapefruit pulp hanging from the ceiling, broken pieces of bottles all over the floor and walls sticky with sugar. The bottles had exploded during the night. Because of misfortunes like these, I always brew the soda in plastic bottles to start with, measure the amount of yeast and soda culture carefully and keep checking the fermenting soda so that it doesn't get over-fermented. When it's finished, I pour the soda through a funnel into glass bottles, with a chopstick in the funnel to prevent foaming when I'm bottling the soda. When the soda is done, I store it in the fridge to stall the fermentation. As the soda slowly continues to ferment even when in the fridge, I never keep it for more than four weeks.

If you follow each recipe exactly there shouldn't be any major disasters with explosions and sugar-sticky walls. But you should always be careful not to over-ferment the soda, and to place it in the fridge to stop fermentation once it's fizzy.

I normally open the bottles carefully over the sink using a bottle opener and if I've brewed in small plastic bottles I unscrew them very slowly.

When you make soda from syrup there is no risk of over-fermentation and explosions, so you can look at it as the slightly 'easier' way to make your own soda. When you are brewing using yeast and soda culture it might be just a bit more 'advanced' but is absolutely not difficult or complicated.

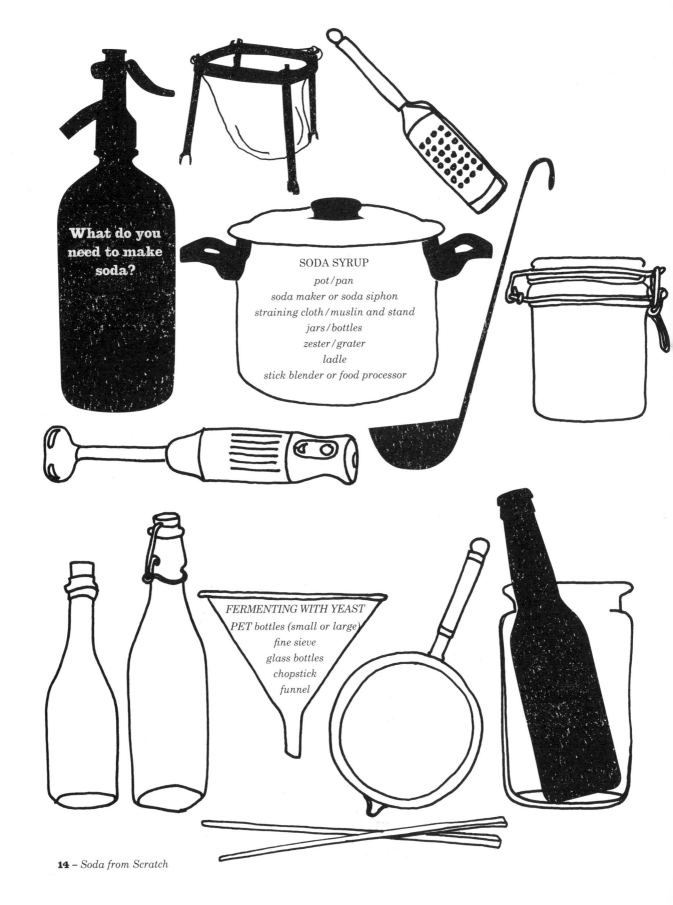

What do you need to make soda?

SODA SYRUP

pot / pan
soda maker or soda siphon
straining cloth / muslin and stand
jars / bottles
zester / grater
ladle
stick blender or food processor

FERMENTING WITH YEAST
PET bottles (small or large)
fine sieve
glass bottles
chopstick
funnel

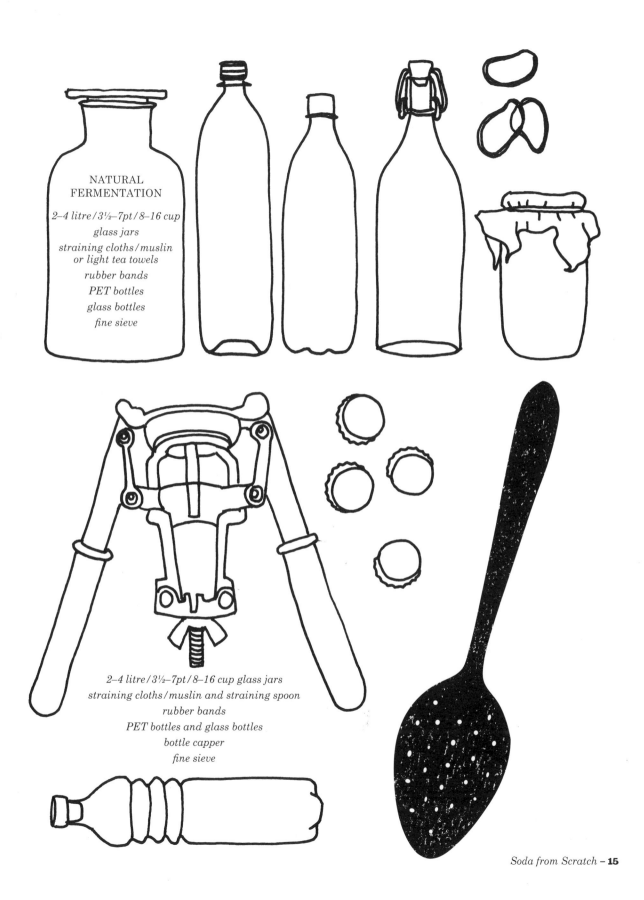

NATURAL
FERMENTATION

*2–4 litre / 3½–7pt / 8–16 cup
glass jars
straining cloths / muslin
or light tea towels
rubber bands
PET bottles
glass bottles
fine sieve*

*2–4 litre / 3½–7pt / 8–16 cup glass jars
straining cloths / muslin and straining spoon
rubber bands
PET bottles and glass bottles
bottle capper
fine sieve*

SUGAR

Sugar is what makes the fermented soda fizzy. The yeast and the bacteria culture eat the sugar and create carbonic acid. You can leave the brew to ferment completely so that almost all the sugar disappears and you're left with a completely dry soda. Some fruit juices, for example sweet strawberries and raspberries, contain quite a lot of natural fructose but can still need an extra dose of sugar to kick-start the fermentation process.

For a sugar-free soda, about 1 tbsp sugar per 1.5 litres / 2½ pints / 6½ cups of liquid is added to get the fermentation started and then berries or other fruits are added for flavour and sweetness, which is eaten by the yeast. The sugar disappears almost completely and the result is a drink with a dry character and sweetness that comes only from fruit. It's also possible to make syrup from coconut sugar or agave syrup, which are regarded as a little more healthy than normal cane and beet sugar.

In the book there are also recipes for herbal infusions (see page 48): these are concentrated herb liquids, almost completely without sugar, which go incredibly well with food. The herbs marry with any herbal notes in the dish and the sensation is similar to drinking green tea with Asian food.

I use all kinds of sugar depending on what character I want in my finished soda.

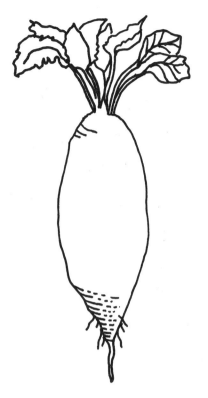

GRANULATED SUGAR

The most common sugar that you can get hold of anywhere, with a neutral colour and taste, granulated sugar is made from sugar beet or sugar cane and gets its white colour through refining (a chemical cleaning process).

Because of the refining process, granulated sugar isn't ideal for making naturally fermented soda. The sugar simply doesn't contain enough natural nutrients to get the bacteria culture started.

Granulated sugar can, on the other hand, be used to make all kinds of soda syrups, lemonade, kombucha and also for soda that is fermented using champagne yeast.

DEMERARA SUGAR

A sugar made from sugar cane, Demerara has been refined to a certain extent, but still has a brown colour and a lot of nutrients that yeast and bacteria culture thrive in. It helps to get the soda fermenting and I've discovered that this is the best sugar to kick-start a soda culture made from ginger. The culture will give a neutral colour and taste to the finished drink, which is a good thing for all kinds of soda production.

Demerara can be found both as slightly larger crystals and as a finer granulated sugar. I often use the finer kind as it's easier to use and dissolves more quickly in liquid than the slightly coarser crystals.

SYRUP AND MOLASSES

Syrup and molasses are by-products from sugar refining, resulting in viscous glucose and fructose and a flavour that tastes nicely of caramel. If you want to cold-mix a soda syrup or lemonade, golden syrup is a good sweetener and will give a pleasant flavour. Syrup can also be used as sweetener for fermented sodas, since the yeast and bacteria culture will thrive in the sweetness of the syrup. I think, however, that it's easier to measure and use dry granulated or cane sugar for fermented soda. This will also give a neutral flavour which is suitable for when you want to enhance the flavours from fruit and berries, otherwise the syrup can easily dominate the flavours in the finished drink. For a richer flavour in your soda – in root beer, cola or juniper berry soda, for example – you can use black treacle or light molasses. It will give the drink a deeper flavour of dried fruit and contribute to a darker colour.

MUSCOVADO SUGAR

This is a raw sugar that is produced from sugar cane. The sugar is almost completely untreated and retains the flavour, nutrients and dark colour, which would otherwise disappear in the refining process. The flavour is fruity and rich with hints of dried fruit, raisins, chocolate and liquorice. The light variety has a mild caramel flavour and the dark one has a strong caramel tone that resembles liquorice and burnt caramel.

As muscovado sugar is rich in flavours and has a unique character, it has a narrower area of usage than cane and granulated sugar. It can be used for spicy soda, for example, cola or juniper berry soda. You can also use light muscovado sugar for Ginger Ale Syrup (page 38); the mild caramel flavour together with the ginger is a good combination. But if you are making a soda culture based on muscovado sugar the soda will be dark in colour and have a rich flavour, which isn't always exactly what you want for raspberry soda, for example. The bacteria will thrive in the dark sugar, but the end result will be different.

HONEY

Honey can be used as a sweetener in syrups and lemonade but won't work for fermented sodas or in kombucha. This is because the yeast bacteria can't find enough sugar in honey, and therefore the fermentation process won't get started.

COCONUT SUGAR

This is extracted from the nectar of the coconut flower and is regarded as being a little better for you than normal sugar made from sugar canes and beets. Coconut sugar has a caramel flavour and a milder sweetness than normal sugar and is nice for using in lemonades and syrups. It's not possible to melt and caramelise coconut sugar, so it can't be used in, for example, Sea Buckthorn Trocadero (page 47) or Cream Soda (page 24). Just like with honey, you can't use coconut sugar for fermented soda or kombucha.

CORN SYRUP

Chemically produced syrup from corn, this is often used in factory-produced soda and pop.

In the US there is currently a big debate going on around corn syrup, as it's regarded as being worse for you than cane sugar and is alleged to have an adverse effect on health. There is no solid proof, but the debate has sparked a flavour-nerd craze for Mexican Fanta and Coca-Cola. Many will happily pay more for Mexican soda in hotels, restaurants and bars as it contains cane sugar.

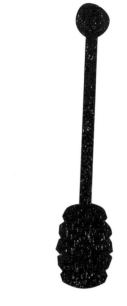

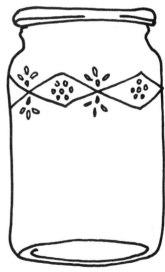

SPICES

When you boil syrup and brew soda you can use a range of spices to develop the right flavour. One example is cola, for which you boil together a spice syrup with cinnamon, star anise, coriander seeds, bitter orange peel, vanilla, ginger, nutmeg, mace... A good deal of spices in just that one type of soda to develop the ultimate cola flavour.

Root beer is the USA's answer to Swedish svagdricka and juniper berry soda. Here, roots, bark and spices are used to develop a rich and unique flavour.

Citric and tartaric acid are used to balance the sweetness in these beverages, as they don't get enough acidity from freshly squeezed citrus fruit. If you add too much citrus juice the sodas will get too watery and the citrus character will be too strong. If citric or tartaric acid is added instead, you get a sharp acidity from just a teaspoon or two.

BITTER ORANGE PEEL
Dried bitter orange peel will give a good citrus flavour and a good amount of bitterness. But use sparingly as its flavour can easily take over.

CARDAMOM
For boiling syrups and adding flavour to other drinks you should use the green cardamom pods. You can add them to the pan for flavour and then strain them off.

CINCHONA BARK
This has long been revered as a source of bitterness. It comes originally from South America and was used as a remedy for malaria. The bark gives Tonic (page 33) its unique, bitter character. Cinchona bark can be found in spice stores, home-brew and health food shops.

CINNAMON
A flavour in many drinks, I use it in Cola (page 40), Christmas Soda (page 102) and The American Southerner's Cinnamon Soda (page 28), for example. Sometimes you want a proper cinnamon flavour and other times a more discreet flavour that matches other spices in the drink. I often use Ceylon cinnamon, which has a fantastic flavour in comparison to the regular cinnamon that you find in the supermarket. You can find Ceylon cinnamon in good food and spice stores.

CORIANDER SEEDS
These can be used for more complex syrup and soda flavours. They really marry with a lot of other flavours from both berries and rich spices.

DANDELION ROOT
An ingredient that is used in, among other things, Root Beer (page 102), but can also be the main star in a soda. In the UK and the US you can often find soda made from dandelion leaves as well as roots. Dandelion root can be found in spice stores, stores specialising in home brewing and in health food stores.

GINGER
Always use fresh root ginger for a clear zingy flavour. Dried ginger can sometimes taste too much of ginger snaps and Christmas spices.

NUTMEG AND MACE
Mace is the lacy net that surrounds the nutmeg seed. It has a milder nutmeg flavour than the seed and can be left to simmer in a syrup without giving a flavour that's too dominant.

SARSAPARILLA BARK
One of the main ingredients in Root Beer (page 102), this can be found in spice stores, stores specialising in home brewing and in health food stores.

SASSAFRAS BARK
Another of the main ingredients in Root Beer (page 102), this can also be found in stores specialising in spices, home brewing and health food.

STAR ANISE
With its mild liquorice flavour star anise has the power to really get the flavours going in a drink. But don't use too much!

VANILLA
When you buy a vanilla pod it's important to make sure that it is soft and a bit wet. If it's dry and hard it has lost some of its fantastic flavour and it will be difficult to scrape out the seeds from the pod.

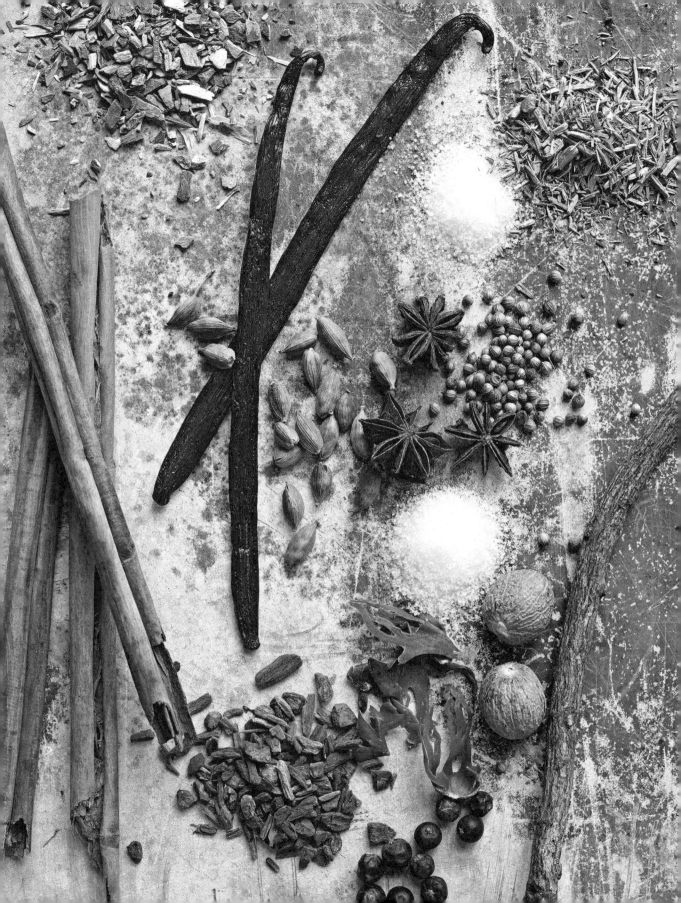

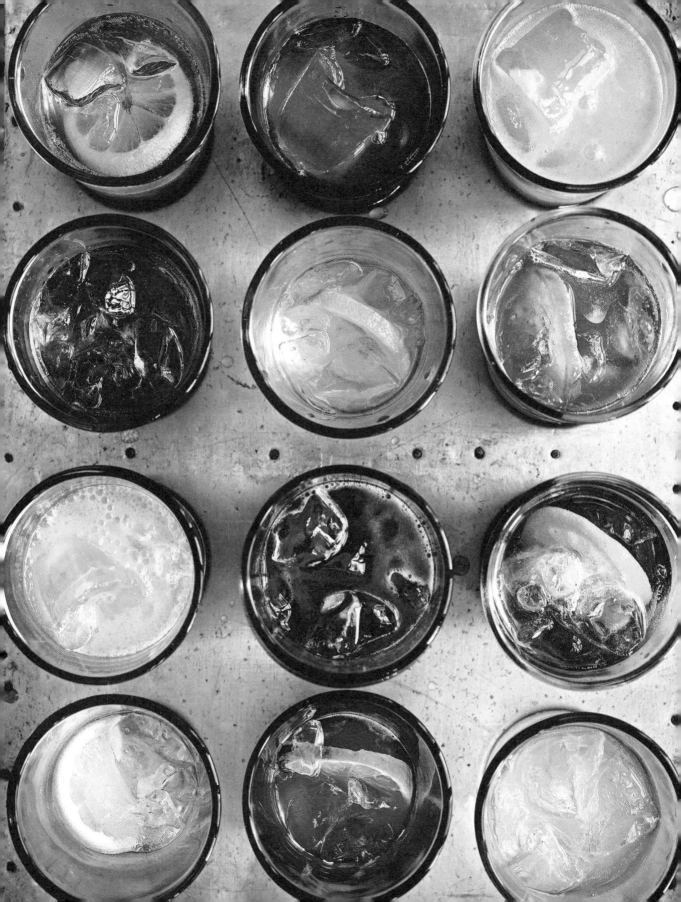

EXTRACTS *and* FOOD COLOURINGS

All my recipes are based on pure ingredients and everything is made from scratch with spices, fruit, berries and herbs to get a soda concentrate, soda or lemonade. No artificially developed extracts or colourings are used to achieve flavours or colours in the drinks. The one exception is bitter almond extract, which is chemically produced to enhance the unique flavour of bitter almond.

FRUIT *and* BERRIES

You can use both fresh and frozen fruit for soda and lemonade. Best is, of course, to use what's in season. If it's summer and the bushes are full of raspberries and strawberries, the best option is to use fresh berries, but if it's autumn and winter you can just use frozen instead.

It's important to let frozen berries thaw thoroughly before using them, as yeast and soda culture don't like the cold. The fermentation process will become difficult to get started and no matter what measures you try the mixture will just stand there without any bubbles appearing. The same thing will happen if it is too warm. Use ingredients at room temperature when preparing soda that needs to ferment.

Citrus fruits are the exception, as they are tastiest during the winter when they're in their best season. But it's not possible to replace freshly squeezed citrus with bottled juice, so do use fresh citrus fruit all the year round when preparing your beverages. This will give you the best flavour, and you'll avoid failed fermentations.

From the SPRINGS *of* HEALTH *to* SUGAR SODA

While making soda obviously began in people's kitchens and progressed to small producers, the classic local soda varieties were pretty much pushed aside in the early twentieth century by the ubiquitous international giants Coca-Cola, Fanta, Pepsi and Sprite.

There were several attempts in various countries to de-throne the factory-produced drinks, and many local specialities began to reappear on the shelves.

But now – at the start of the twenty-first century – a new fizzy drinks revolution has spread not just over my home country of Sweden but throughout the UK, Europe and in other parts of the Western world. Factory-produced soda and fizzy drinks from small micro-breweries using natural fermentation processes and often organic ingredients are increasingly available and growing in popularity. The soda has returned, and preferably it should be naturally produced. Italian blood orange soda, British sparkling lemonade, German cola and kombucha are only a few of the exciting products that you'll now find on the shelves.

The next step, of course, is to experiment with recreating that tasty orange or creamy soda at home in your kitchen.

American SODA FOUNTAINS

Carbonated water mixed with flavoured syrup is the original drink that kick-started soda production in the US in the late nineteenth century.

During Prohibition, when it became illegal to consume alcoholic drinks, soda played an important role. Soda bars started to pop up, and soda fountains were introduced, often in connection with drug stores and pharmacies. People could go there to get a bubbling soda on tap, where so-called soda jerks stood and pumped carbonated water from the taps and mixed it with ice and their own range of flavoured syrups. Incidentally, the word jerk came from the jerking movement that was used to pump up the water.

The reason for connecting the soda fountains with pharmacies was to make the soda water appear just as healthy as water from natural mineral springs that bubbled up straight from the ground.

American soda fountains became social junctions where everyone could go, young or old, and grab a soda and something to eat. Soda jerks developed new soda drinks —such as egg cream, ice cream soda and floats – the common factor being that they were all carbonated and cold.

SODA SYRUP

Soda syrup is mixed with carbonated water, either from a soda maker, siphon or from bought bottled sparkling water. You should avoid the latter as much as you can as there's excellent water in the tap that can be carbonated with carbon dioxide cartridges. This is the classic way to make soda and is used in today's fizzy drinks production. You produce a sweet concentrated syrup base, which is then mixed with carbonated water and the result is a flavoured fizzy drink.

Syrup can be cold-mixed or boiled. The boiled version keeps for longer and takes on more flavour and character. The cold-mixed is easy to whip up when you want flavoured sparkling water quickly.

It's possible to cook syrup from fruit, berries, spices, herbs and bark. They all have the same base – water and sugar. To make sure it doesn't get too sweet I always add some element of acidity, either in the form of freshly squeezed citrus fruit or tartaric or citric acid.

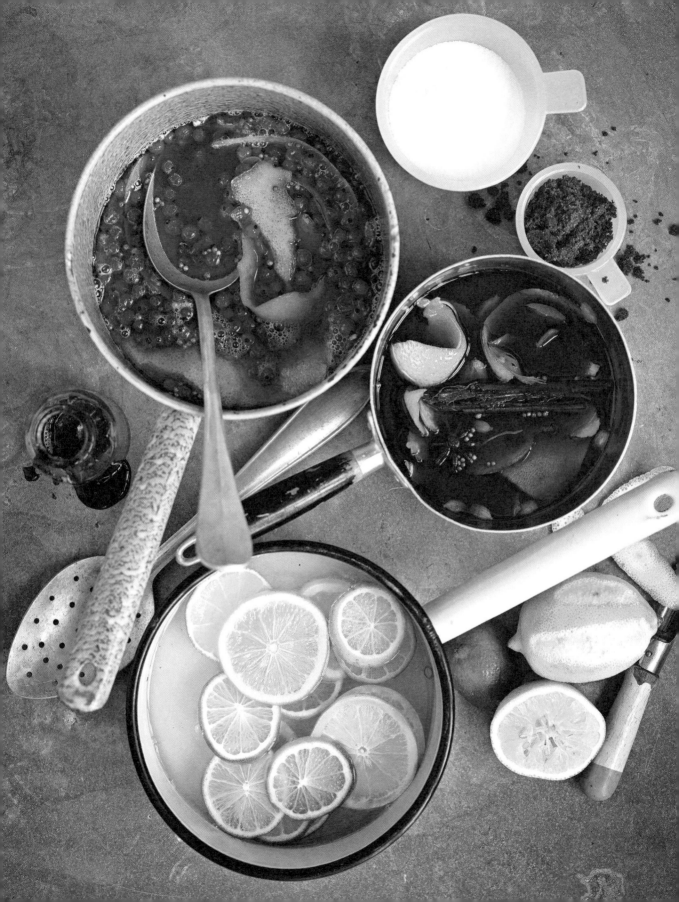

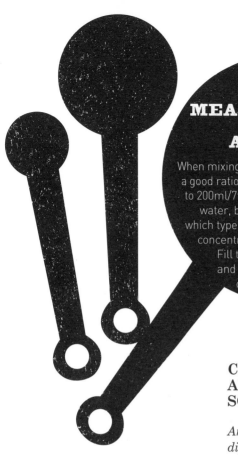

MEASUREMENTS *and* AMOUNTS

When mixing syrup with carbonated water a good ratio is normally 1–1½ tbsp syrup to 200ml/7fl oz/scant 1 cup carbonated water, but it varies depending on which type of syrup you've got and how concentrated you want your soda. Fill the glass with ice first and then stir in syrup and carbonated water.

STORAGE

Soda syrups should be stored in the fridge in airtight jars or bottles. Depending on what the syrup contains it has a shelf life of 4 weeks to 3 months. Syrups containing fruit and berries, that will therefore ferment, keep fresh in the fridge for 4–6 weeks. Spice syrups, for example cola, tonic and ginger ale, can keep fresh for up to 3 months in the fridge. Open the jar and smell the syrup – if it has a fresh smell and there are no bubbles from fermentation you can go ahead and use it. Store in several small jars or bottles and they'll keep for longer unopened.

CREAM SODA – AMERICAN SUGAR SODA

American sugar soda is quite different from its European counterpart. The Swedish version is sweet with hints of fruit and acidity, while the American version is vanilla-sweet and the colour is light brown because the sugar is caramelised before the syrup is boiled with the vanilla pod. There are plenty of stories about the origin of the name, since the drink doesn't have anything to do with cream. Some say it's because earlier recipes used cream of tartar. I think a better explanation is that the flavour is reminiscent of the sugary crust on a creamy crème brûlée. The American version is a little too sweet for my liking, so in my recipe I balance out the sweetness with freshly squeezed lemon juice.

About 1 litre/1¾ pints/4⅓ cups
750g/1lb 10oz/heaped 3¾ cups granulated sugar
500ml/17fl oz/generous 2 cups water
½ vanilla pod, cut open and seeds scraped out
100ml/3½fl oz/scant ½ cup freshly squeezed lemon juice (about 1½–2 lemons)

Put the sugar in a pan and melt over a medium heat until golden and caramelised. Don't stir the sugar, instead shake the pan so that you get an even caramelisation. If you stir, the sugar will melt unevenly and large sugar crystals will get stuck on the spoon.

Remove from the heat and add the water and vanilla seeds. The sugar will get a 'shock' from the cold water, so keep your face away so it doesn't splash you. Simmer until the sugar has dissolved. Cover and leave to cool for 1 hour. Add the lemon juice, then strain and bottle in sterilised bottles. Store the soda in a cool place.

RASPBERRY SYRUP

Simple flavours – raspberry and lemon. Mix together with carbonated water to taste.

About 1 litre/1¾ pints/4⅓ cups
650g/1lb 7oz raspberries
675g/1½lb/3⅓ cups granulated sugar
350ml/12fl oz/1½ cups water
150ml/¼ pint/⅔ cup freshly squeezed lemon juice (2–3 lemons)
½ tsp citric acid

Boil the raspberries, sugar and water together in a pan. Remove from the heat, cover with a clean tea towel and leave to cool.

Stir in the lemon juice and citric acid. Strain through a straining cloth or muslin and bottle in sterilised glass bottles.

GRAPEFRUIT SODA

Fresh and bitter. There is a lot of bitterness in the white pith of the grapefruit so the more white pith, the more bitter the syrup. Do try this with red grapes as well. The flavour will get a little more fragrant, which can be nice, especially with a slice of lemon in an ice-filled glass.

About 1 litre/1¾ pints/4⅓ cups
zest of 3 grapefruits
300ml/½ pint/1¼ cups freshly
   squeezed grapefruit juice
   (about 3 grapefruits)
100ml/3½fl oz/scant ½ cup water
100ml/3½fl oz/scant ½ cup freshly
   squeezed lemon juice
   (1½–2 lemons)
1 tsp citric acid
400g/14oz/2 cups granulated sugar
1 pinch of sea salt

Rinse the grapefruits thoroughly, then peel them using a peeling knife or a vegetable peeler. Put the zest to one side.

Mix together the grapefruit juice, water, lemon juice, citric acid, sugar and salt in a pan. Bring to the boil, then remove from the heat. Stir in the grapefruit zest. Leave to cool

and steep for about 1 hour.

Strain though a straining cloth or muslin. Bottle in sterilised glass bottles, then store in the fridge.

RHUBARB, LIME & LEMONGRASS SODA

Pink or red rhubarb will make this soda a beautiful light pink, but you can also use rhubarb that has more of a green tinge. The colour of the soda will be slightly duller, but it will have a very nice and slightly sharp taste.

About 1 litre/1¾ pints/4⅓ cups
1 lemongrass stalk
500g/1lb 2oz rhubarb, chopped
400g/14oz/2 cups granulated sugar
400ml/14fl oz/1¾ cups water
200ml/7fl oz/scant 1 cup freshly
   squeezed lime juice
   (about 6 limes)
½ tsp citric acid

Bash the lemongrass stalk using the back of a knife or a pestle. Shred the lemongrass and boil together with the rhubarb, sugar and water in a pan until the rhubarb is soft. Remove from the heat and leave to cool covered with a clean tea towel.

Stir in the lime juice and citric acid. Strain firstly through a fine sieve and then through a straining cloth or muslin. Bottle the syrup in sterilised glass bottles and store in the fridge.

LEMONADE SYRUP

The lemonade you buy in the UK is similar to Swedish fruit soda: a fizzy, transparent soda with a sweet and slightly fruity acidic flavour. It's used to mix the summer punch, Pimm's, with a slice of lime – refreshing on a warm day – or is added to beer to make Bitter Shandy (see page 74).

About 600ml/1 pint/generous
   2½ cups
350g/12oz/1¾ cups granulated
   sugar
500ml/17fl oz/generous 2 cups
   water
3 tbsp freshly squeezed lemon
   juice (about ½ lemon)
1½ tsp citric acid

Boil the sugar and water together in a pan until the sugar has dissolved. Remove from the heat and stir in the lemon juice and citric acid. Leave to cool. Bottle in sterilised bottles and store in the fridge.

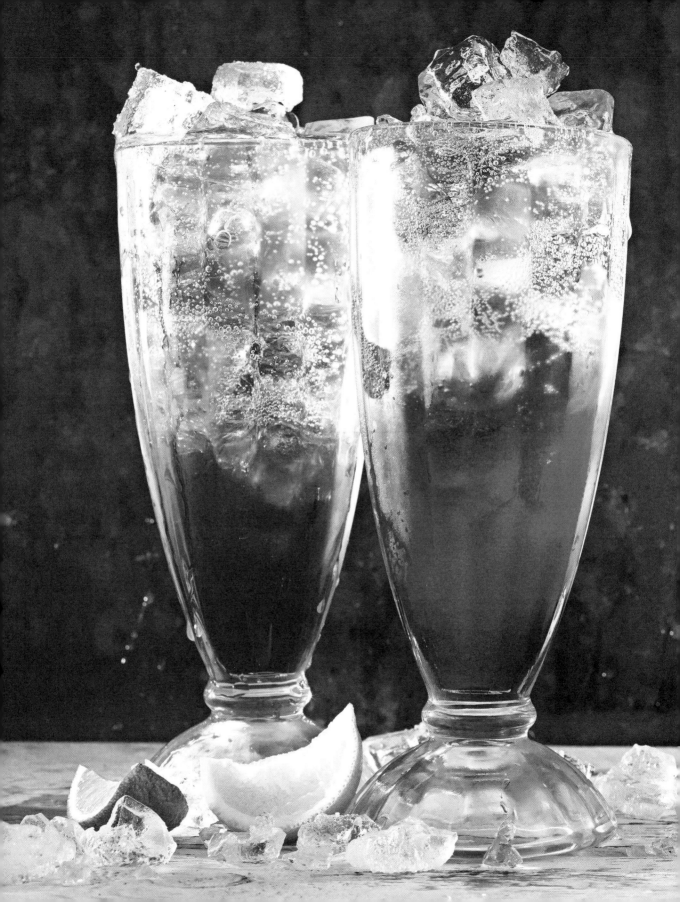

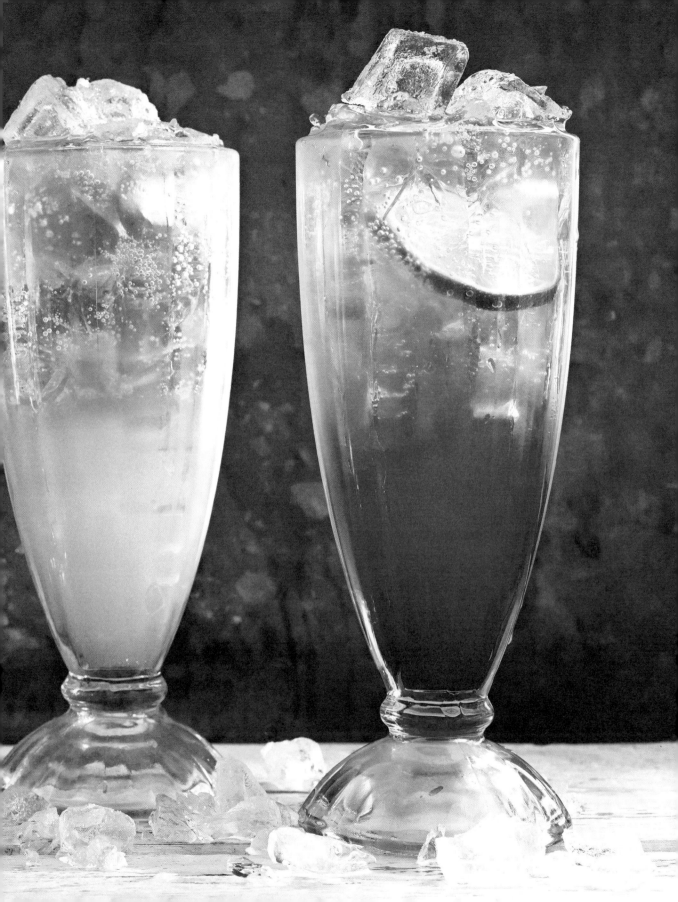

THE AMERICAN SOUTHERNER'S CINNAMON SODA

In the southern parts of the US, where meat is smoked for hours and served up on trays with mac 'n' cheese, fried beans and coleslaw, cinnamon soda is often enjoyed with food. Unfortunately, unnatural food colourings and flavouring extracts are often used to get that bright red colour and spiciness.

This recipe is a variation on that soda. To get the characteristic red colour, hibiscus flower is used, or flor de Jamaica, as they call it in Mexico. Dried hibiscus flower can be found in spice stores and health food stores.

If you love the cinnamon flavour, serve it with an extra cinnamon stick in each glass.

About 400ml/14fl oz/1¾ cups
1 pomegranate
135g/4¾oz/⅔ cup granulated or
    Demerara sugar
600ml/1 pint/2½ cups clear apple
    juice (not cloudy)
8 cinnamon sticks
½ tbsp dried hibiscus flower
1½ tsp citric acid

Deseed the pomegranate. Melt the sugar in a pan until golden brown. Remove from the heat.

Add the apple juice to the pan – it will splash because of the heat from the sugar, so be careful! The sugar will set and line the bottom of the pan. Lift it carefully with a fork or spoon so that it dissolves in the liquid.

Blend the cinnamon sticks into a coarse powder in a food processor or pestle and mortar. Add the powder to the pan together with hibiscus flower and citric acid. Simmer without a lid for about 30 minutes. Cover with a lid and leave to cool.

Strain through a straining cloth or muslin and bottle in a sterilised bottle. Leave to cool, then store in the fridge.

STICK FRIES

Like a mix between fries and crisps, these crispy potato sticks have an onion flavour.

Serves 4
500g/1lb 2oz floury potatoes, such
    as Maris Piper
1-1.5 litres/1¾-2½ pints/
    4⅓-6½ cups deep-frying oil,
    such as rapeseed oil
½ tsp onion powder
1 tsp salt flakes
flavoured mayonnaise (see right),
    to serve (optional)

Slice the potatoes thinly, then shred into thin sticks. Place them in ice-cold water and leave in the fridge for about 1 hour. Drain off the water and leave the potato sticks to dry on a clean tea towel. Leave in a cold place for a further 30 minutes.

Heat the oil to 160°C/315°F. Deep-fry the potato sticks in batches until golden brown and crispy. Take them out of the pan with a slotted spoon and leave to drain on kitchen paper. Toss with the onion powder and salt while still warm. Enjoy the fries on their own or dipped in flavoured mayonnaise.

CORIANDER MAYONNAISE

About 250ml/9fl oz/generous 1 cup
2½ egg yolks
1½ tbsp freshly squeezed lime
    juice, plus extra to taste
2 tsp ground coriander
25g/1oz/½ cup chopped fresh
    coriander
1 garlic clove, finely grated
250ml/9fl oz/generous 1 cup
    rapeseed oil
salt

Mix together the egg yolks, lime juice, ground and fresh coriander and garlic in a blender. With the motor running, gradually blend in the oil, one drop at a time, until you get a thick, green mayonnaise. Season to taste with salt and, if needed, a little more lime.

CHILLI MAYONNAISE

About 250ml/9fl oz/generous 1 cup
2 egg yolks
1½ tbsp white wine vinegar
1 tbsp Japanese soy sauce
½ garlic clove, finely grated
2 tbsp sriracha sauce (Thai chilli
    sauce)
250ml/9fl oz/generous 1 cup
    rapeseed oil
salt
a dash of chilli sauce (optional)

Whisk together the egg yolks, vinegar, soy sauce, garlic and sriracha sauce in a bowl.

Gradually whisk in the oil, one drop at a time, until you get a thick, creamy mayonnaise. Season to taste with salt, more vinegar and a dash of chilli sauce, if needed.

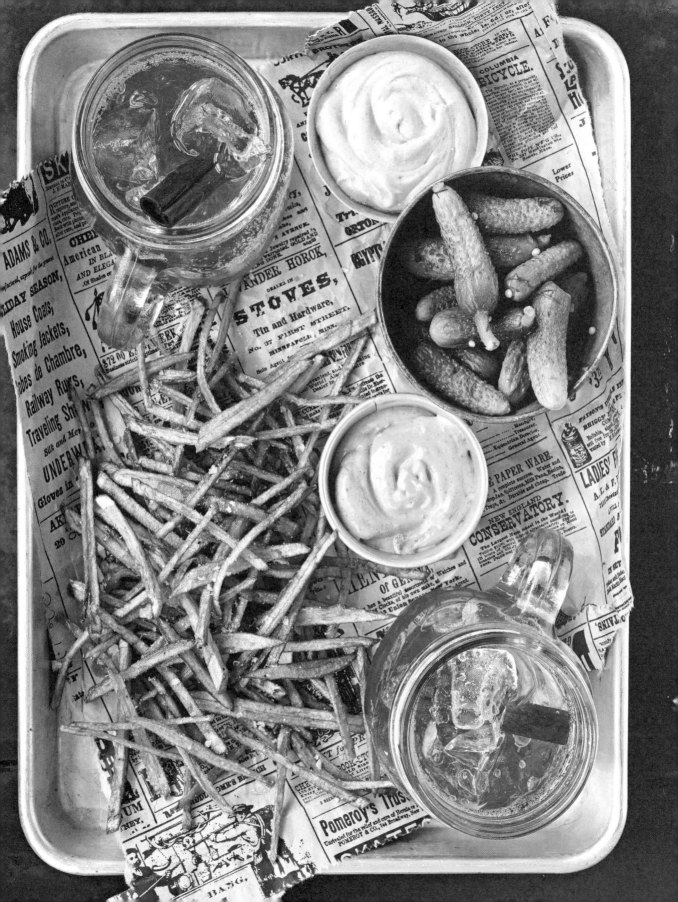

EXOTIC PASSION SYRUP

Passion fruit, pineapple and lime. The syrup will be tastiest if you use a juicer, but it works fine with shop-bought pineapple juice too. If you use the latter, you can reduce the sugar by 50g / 1¾oz / ¼ cup.

About 500ml/17fl oz/
    generous 2 cups
100g/3½oz passion fruit flesh
    (about 5–6 passion fruits)
1½ tsp citric acid
500ml/17fl oz/generous 2 cups
    pineapple juice
300g/10½oz/1½ cups granulated
    sugar
100ml/3½fl oz/scant ½ cup freshly
    squeezed lime juice (about
    3 limes)

Halve the passion fruits and scrape out the flesh into a pan. Add the citric acid, pineapple juice and sugar. Bring to the boil, then leave to reduce for about 10 minutes.

Add the lime juice and leave to cool.

Strain through a straining cloth or muslin or a fine sieve. Bottle in sterilised bottles and store in a cool place.

DRAGON FRUIT SYRUP

Here the syrup doesn't have to be boiled, instead it's cold-mixed and then blended, getting its bright pink colour from the peel of the fruit. Because of the starch from the fruit, the consistency of the mixed soda can seem quite thick, but with the fresh acidity breaking through it really becomes a refreshing drink. Serve with lots of ice.

About 200ml/7fl oz/scant 1 cup
½ dragon fruit (pitaya)
100ml/3½fl oz/scant ½ cup freshly
    squeezed lime juice (about
    3 limes)
3–4 tbsp clear honey

Cut off the outer peel from the dragon fruit, but keep the inner pink peel. Cut the fruit into pieces and blend into a purée using a stick blender. Mix with the lime juice and honey.

Fill a glass with ice and mix together the syrup and some carbonated water.

PLANTAIN CRISPS

Thinly sliced, deep-fried plantain makes delicious crunchy crisps. No, you can't replace the plantain with banana! A banana will mostly turn into a mush if deep-fried.

Serves 4
2–3 plantains
1–1.5 litres/1¾–2½ pints/
    4⅓–6½ cups deep-frying oil,
    such as rapeseed oil
salt

Peel the plantains using a peeling knife or a vegetable peeler. Slice into thin diagonal slices, about 1–2mm/¹⁄₁₆in thick.

Heat the oil to 180°C/350°F. Deep-fry in batches for about 2–3 minutes until the slices have turned into crunchy crisps. Drain on kitchen paper.

Toss the crisps in some salt while still warm, then leave to cool before serving.

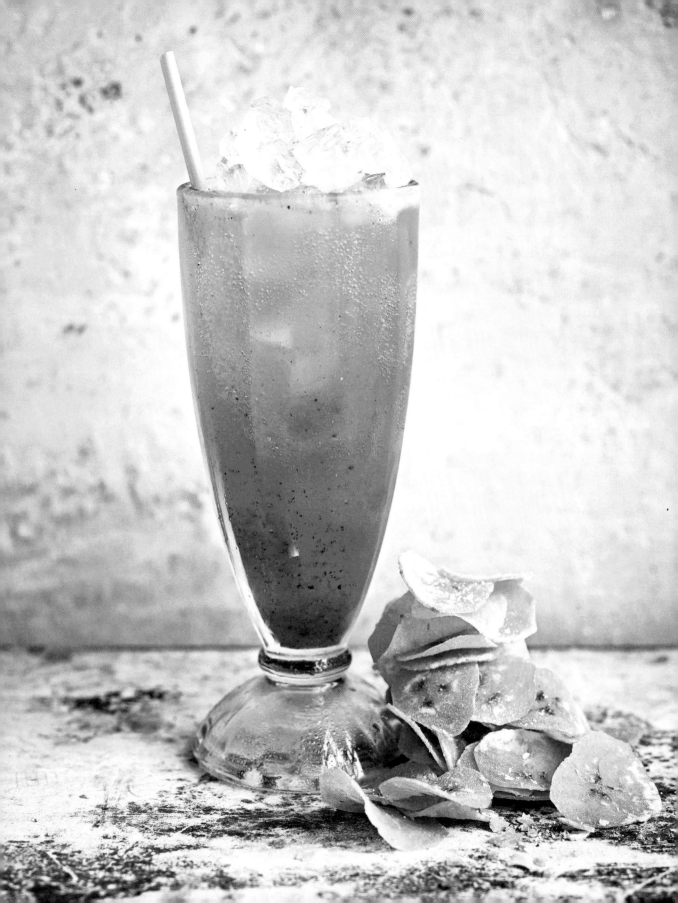

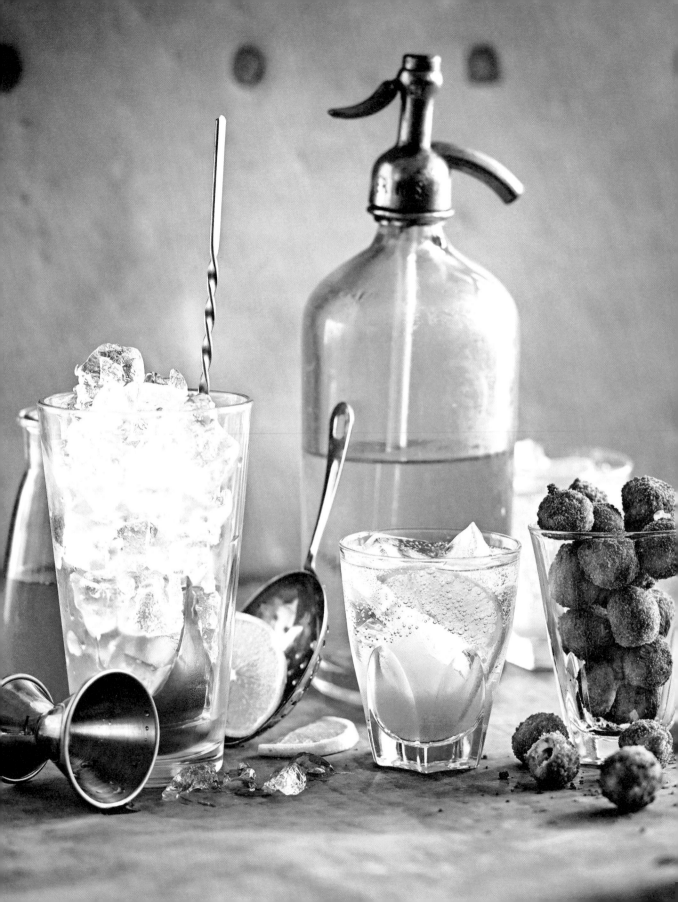

TONIC SYRUP

Tonic is nice to drink just as it is in a glass with lemon and ice, but there's nothing that better suits a relaxed summer holiday than an afternoon G&T. We're dealing here with two, or at most three ingredients, if you count the lemon, so any lazy holiday-maker can quickly mix together a proper gin cocktail. With homemade tonic in the fridge you'll add some extra finesse to this simple drink.

To make tonic syrup you don't need that many ingredients, but you'll have to be careful to get the quantities right for this bitter concentrate. The bitterness comes from cinchona bark, which originated in Peru and was spread across the world by the Spanish colonisers when they saw that the Indians used a brew made from the bark to protect themselves against malaria.

This remedy later became a saviour for the British colonisers who had to gulp down the bitter brew while travelling around building their empire. It was probably a real genius of a soldier who came up with the idea to mix the brew with some sugar, soda water and gin to keep healthy and in good spirits. The G&T was born!

About 400ml/14fl oz/1¾ cups
500ml/17fl oz/generous 2 cups water
200g/7oz/1 cup granulated sugar
150g/5½oz/¾ cup Demerara sugar
1½ pieces of cinchona bark, finely ground to a powder
4 allspice berries, crushed
3 juniper berries, crushed
1 lemongrass stalk, shredded
grated zest of ½ orange
grated zest of ½ lemon
grated zest of ½ lime
2 tsp citric acid
a pinch of salt

Bring all the ingredients to the boil in a pan, then leave to simmer for about 15 minutes. Leave to cool, then strain through a straining cloth or muslin. Store in a cool place.

Mix about 1 tbsp syrup with 200ml/7fl oz/scant 1 cup soda water for a perfectly bitter and refreshing tonic.

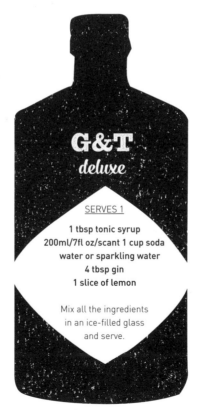

G&T
deluxe

SERVES 1

1 tbsp tonic syrup
200ml/7fl oz/scant 1 cup soda water or sparkling water
4 tbsp gin
1 slice of lemon

Mix all the ingredients in an ice-filled glass and serve.

DEEP-FRIED OLIVES

This is the ultimate snack to go with gin and tonic or a classic dry martini. You can vary the filling – chilli, pimiento, lemon or anchovy all work well. The olives are best when freshly fried, but will keep crisp for a few hours.

Serves 4
600ml/1 pint/generous 2 cups deep-frying oil, such as rapeseed oil
200g/7oz/2 cups pitted green olives, filled with lemon, anchovy, pimento or a filling of your choice
55g/2oz/½ cup plain flour
1 egg, beaten
80g/2¾oz/1 cup dried breadcrumbs

Heat the oil to 180°C/350°F. Drain the olives and coat them in flour. Dip the olives first in the beaten egg and then in the breadcrumbs.

Deep-fry in the hot oil until crispy and golden brown, about 2–3 minutes. Leave to drain on a piece of kitchen paper. Serve warm or at room temperature.

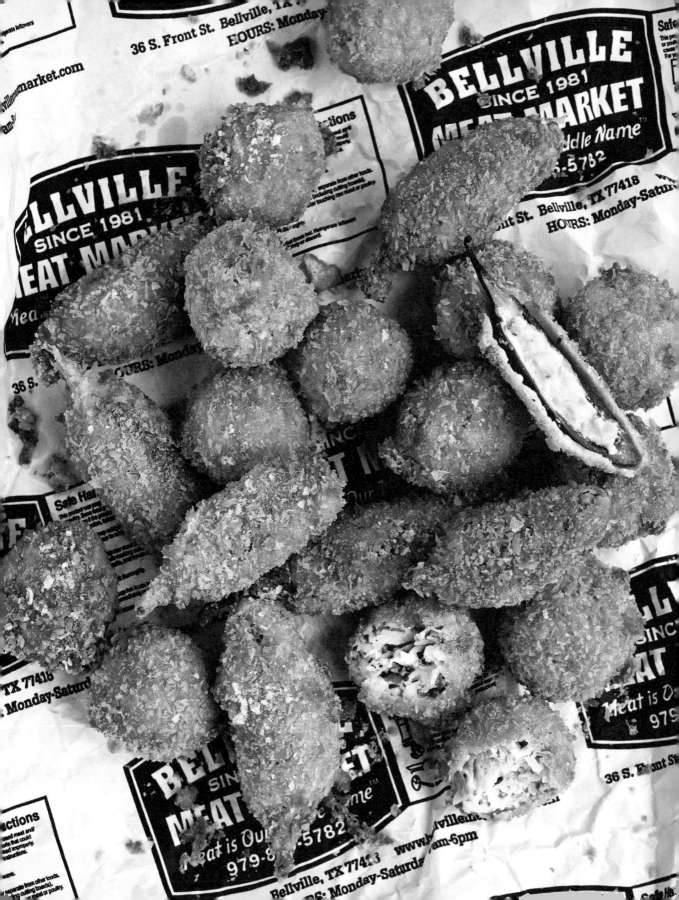

POPPERS

Yes, I love deep-fried food. There's nothing as good as things freshly fried, crispy, crunchy and flaky. If they also contain melted cheese, I'm completely sold. Poppers, small croquettes, are perfect as snacks for an evening of mingling – something fairly substantial to eat in between drinks, bubbles and soda. The favourite is definitely poppers with sauerkraut, bacon and cheese – an unbeatable combination.

JALAPEÑO & PADRÓN POPPERS

A classic – Cheddar and a good amount of heat from the jalapeño chilli pepper. For a change, you could fill the small green peppers, pimiento de Padrón, with the mixture and deep-fry. They've got a good bitterness, without as much heat – unless you're unlucky and get the occasional hot one – some say it's one in ten, others one in 20 or one in 100.

Makes 12

50g/1¾oz cream cheese
100g/3½oz Cheddar cheese, grated
12 jalapeño or pimiento de
   Padrón
1–1.5 litres/1¾–2½ pints/
   4⅓–6½ cups deep-frying oil,
   such as rapeseed oil
120g/4¼oz/scant 1 cup plain flour
2 eggs, beaten
85g/3oz/1¾ cups panko
   breadcrumbs
salt flakes

Mix the cream cheese and Cheddar to a paste. Make a cut lengthways in the jalapeños and carefully scrape out the seeds. Fill with the cheese mixture using small spoon.

Heat the oil to 180°C/350°F in a deep-fryer or in a large pan.

Sprinkle the jalapeños with some water and roll them in flour. Dip first into the beaten egg and then in panko.

Deep-fry until golden brown and crispy, about 2–3 minutes. Take out with a slotted spoon and leave to drain on a piece of kitchen paper. Sprinkle with salt flakes to serve.

SAUERKRAUT, BACON & CHEESE POPPERS

Cabbage, bacon, cheese, cumin and caraway. Try swapping the cabbage for kimchi and mix with Cheddar – also extremely tasty! If you don't have spiced cheese you can use Cheddar and add ½ tsp caraway seeds and ½ tsp whole cumin seeds.

Makes 20

140g/5oz bacon, finely diced
250g/9oz sauerkraut
150g/5oz spiced cheese, coarsely
   grated
3 eggs
85g/3oz/1¾ cups panko
   breadcrumbs
120g/4¼oz/scant 1 cup plain flour
1–1.5 litres/1¾–2½ pints/
   4⅓–6½ cups deep-frying oil,
   such as rapeseed oil
salt flakes

Fry the bacon until crisp in a dry pan. Drain on kitchen paper.

Quickly whiz together the sauerkraut, bacon and cheese in a food processor. The filling should be chopped, not turned into a purée. Mix with 1 egg, 40g/1½oz/½ cup of the panko and 2 tbsp of the flour. Leave to absorb the liquid for about 15 minutes in the fridge.

Heat the oil to 180°C/350°F.

Shape the filling into 20 equally sized balls and roll them carefully in the remaining flour, then the beaten egg, and finally the panko.

Deep-fry for 3–5 minutes until golden brown with a crispy crust. Sprinkle with salt flakes.

CRAB POPPERS

Luxury poppers with red king crab. Nice to munch on with ginger beer, barley water or lemon soda.

Makes about 12

250g/9oz meat from red king crab
   (about 3 legs), coarsely chopped
25g/10z/½ cup chives, chopped
3 eggs
85g/3oz/1¾ cups panko
   breadcrumbs
120g/4¼oz/scant 1 cup plain flour
salt and black pepper
1–1.5 litres/1¾–2½ pints/
   4⅓–6½ cups deep-frying oil,
   such as rapeseed oil
salt flakes

Mix the crabmeat with the chives, 1 egg, 40g/1½oz/½ cup of the panko, 2 tbsp of the flour, and salt and pepper. Shape the filling into balls. Coat in flour, then in the remaining beaten egg and finally in panko.

Heat the oil to 180°C/350°F and deep-fry the balls until golden brown and crisp, about 1–2 minutes. Sprinkle with salt flakes to taste.

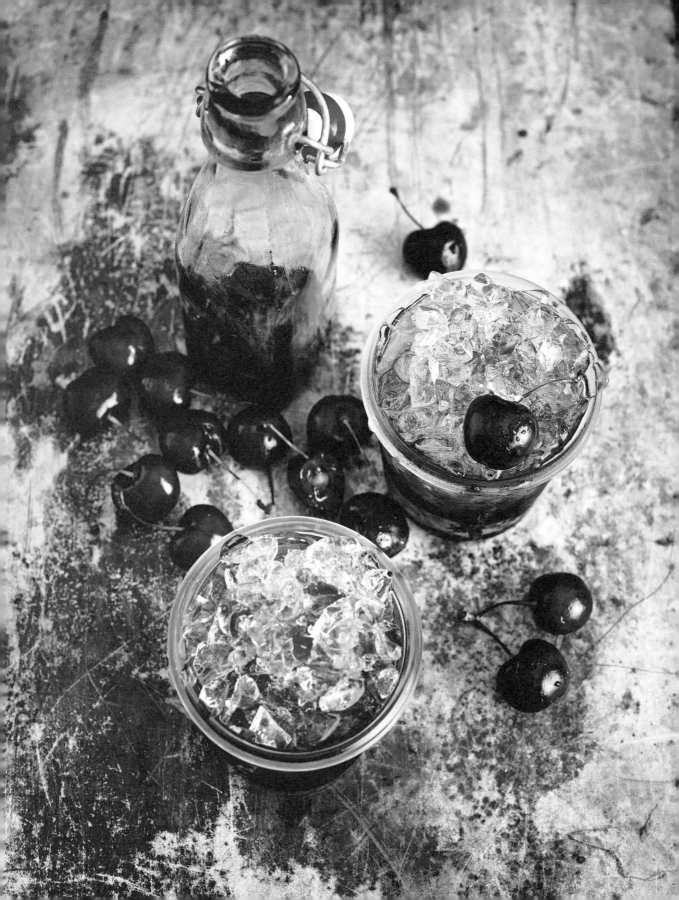

ROB'S FAVOURITE CHERRY SODA

Amaretto liqueur, tiramisu, almond biscotti, chocolate and cherry soda – none of these would be the same without the taste of bitter almond! It's what makes Cherry Coke and Dr. Pepper taste slightly artificially but nicely of cherries. The unique flavour sits in the stones of peaches, nectarines, apricots, plums and cherries. When fermenting fruit wine – for example, cherry or plum wine – the stones are included, either crushed or whole. That's what gives the drink the lovely flavour of bitter almond. Since soda syrup is neither fermented or boiled for very long, bitter almond extract is used in this recipe to get the right flavour.

About 8 litres/14 pints/8½ quarts
500g/1lb 2oz cherries, rinsed
   and pitted
225g/8oz/1¼ cups Demerara sugar
300ml/½ pint/1¼ cups water
½ tsp citric acid
150ml/¼ pint/scant ⅔ cup freshly
   squeezed lemon juice
   (about 2–3 lemons)
finely grated zest of 1 lemon
scant ¼ tsp bitter almond extract
a pinch of salt
cocktail cherries, to garnish

Bring the cherries, sugar, water and citric acid to the boil in a pan. Leave to simmer gently for about 20 minutes until the cherries break apart and the syrup goes red and thickens.

Remove from the heat and stir in the lemon juice, lemon zest, bitter almond extract and salt. Leave to cool. Strain through a straining cloth or muslin and bottle in a sterilised glass bottle. Store in the fridge.

Mix together with soda water and ice and top with a cocktail cherry to serve.

Cherry ice cream
Make use of the cherries left over from the straining. Run them in an ice-cream maker together with a batch of Vanilla Ice Cream (see page 108). Very nice!

FRESH GINGER & RASPBERRY SYRUP

Fresh flavour with a peppery sting from the ginger. This syrup is freshly squeezed and cold-mixed and won't keep for as long as other syrups. Store it in the fridge and drink within two days. Mix about 2½ tbsp syrup with 200ml / 7fl oz / scant 1 cup carbonated water.

About 400ml/14fl oz/1¾ cups
135g/4¾oz/ ⅔ cup Demerara sugar
250ml/9fl oz/generous 1 cup water
1½ tsp citric acid
300g/10½oz fresh root ginger
100g/3½oz raspberries

Boil the sugar, 150ml/¼ pint/scant ⅔ cup of the water and the citric acid together to make a simple syrup. Leave to cool.

Peel and run the ginger though a juicer, you should end up with about 150ml/ ¼ pint/scant ⅔ cup ginger juice. Mix the juice with the syrup, the remaining water and the raspberries. Blend with a stick blender, then strain through a fine sieve. Store in a cool place.

BITTER SODA WITH GRAPEFRUIT & RED CURRANTS

Bitter drinks are a bit of a summer favourite. Campari and Aperol with soda water are refreshing and the bitter after-taste is delicious with salty crisps or nuts.

My version of the Italian favourite is a proper bitter syrup with a flavour of grapefruit and a lovely freshness from summer-picked, slightly sour, red currants. If you're feeling like a stronger drink, you can mix it with sparkling wine to make a delicious summer spritzer.

About 700ml/24fl oz/3 cups
3 grapefruits
350ml/12fl oz/1½ cups freshly squeezed grapefruit juice (about 3–4 grapefruits)
200ml/7fl oz/scant 1 cup water
225g/8oz red currants
1 tsp whole coriander seeds
1½ tsp tartaric acid
350g/12oz/1¾ cups granulated sugar
a pinch of salt

Peel the grapefruits using a vegetable peeler. Don't worry about not including any white parts. Instead you can cut the peel into chunky slices to include the white pith underneath the skin, as it will give a bitter character to the syrup.

Mix together the grapefruit peel and juice, water, red currants, coriander seeds, tartaric acid, sugar and salt in a large pan. Bring to the boil and simmer without a lid for about 10 minutes. Leave to cool covered with a lid.

Strain through a straining cloth or muslin and bottle in small sterilised bottles. Keep in the fridge.

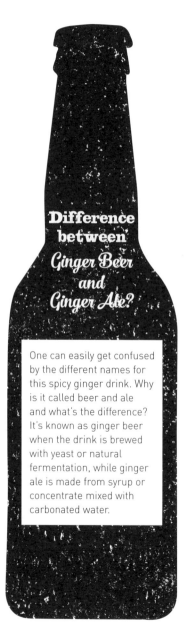

Difference between Ginger Beer and Ginger Ale?

One can easily get confused by the different names for this spicy ginger drink. Why is it called beer and ale and what's the difference? It's known as ginger beer when the drink is brewed with yeast or natural fermentation, while ginger ale is made from syrup or concentrate mixed with carbonated water.

GINGER ALE SYRUP

A glass filled with ginger ale is tasty just on its own, but a cocktail made from homemade ginger ale is considerably nicer than one made from the shop-bought variety. This syrup has a really good balance between the kick from the ginger, the sweetness from the sugar and the acidity from the citric acid.

About 800ml/28fl oz/3½ cups
200g/7oz fresh root ginger, chopped
500ml/17fl oz/generous 2 cups water
finely grated zest of 1 lemon
1 tsp citric acid
a large pinch of salt
200g/7oz/1 cup light muscovado sugar
200g/7oz/1 cup Demerara sugar

Blend the ginger in a food processor. (You don't have to peel it if it's rinsed thoroughly.) Blend properly until it's almost turned into a purée.

Bring the water, ginger, lemon zest, citric acid and salt to the boil. Leave to simmer gently for about 5 minutes.

Add the sugar and stir so that it dissolves in the liquid. Remove from the heat and leave to cool, covered with a lid or muslin.

Strain through a straining cloth or muslin. Bottle in a sterilised glass bottle and store in the fridge.

Mix together with ice and carbonated water.

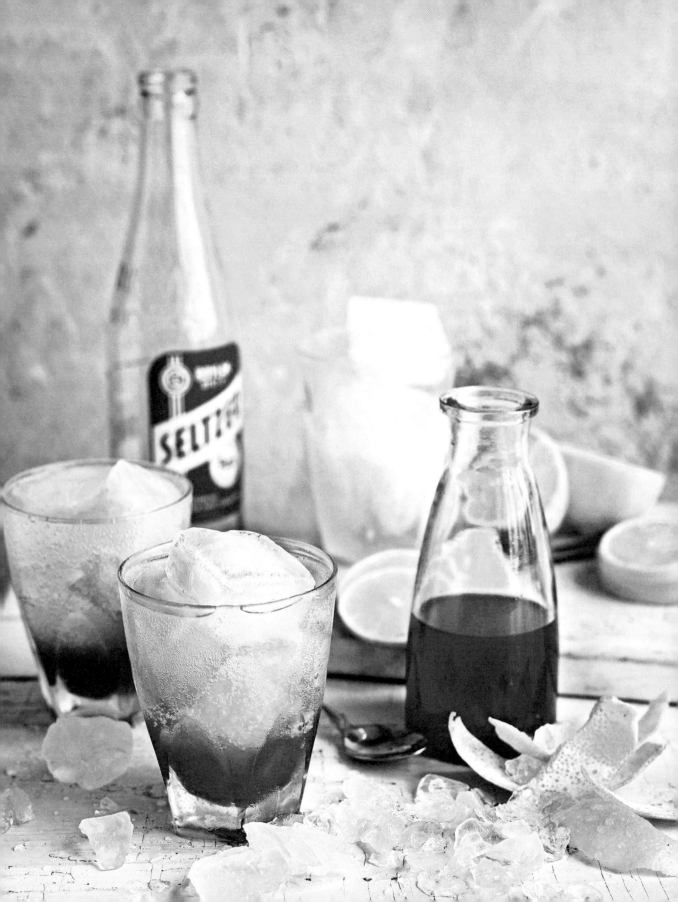

COLA SYRUP

The road to the perfect cola is long. Should you use nutmeg, cinnamon, ginger, vanilla, star anise, muscovado, molasses or perhaps liquorice root? You want to achieve that perfect balance between the spicy, the sweet and the sour.

After many attempts I eventually gave up and instead aimed to produce a drink with a similar cola flavour to the ice-lollies from my childhood. My version is slightly spicier and is quite acidic from lemon and lime.

Since the first bottle of Coca-Cola was mixed at the end of the 19th century there have been many attempts to imitate and get that unique flavour right. In Sweden, Cuba-Cola was developed and launched in the summer of 1953. Cola drinks had been banned before then, as they contained phosphoric acid and caffeine. When the ban was lifted, the Cuba-Cola came out on the Swedish market, but only three months after the launch, Coca-Cola was introduced in Sweden and was a major competitor. It's said, however, that the Swedish drink became more popular during the 1960s and 70s when the leftist movement spread across the country.

About 1 litre/1¾ pints/4⅓ cups
STEP 1
400ml/14fl oz/1¾ cups water
400ml/14fl oz/1¾ cups clear
   apple juice (not cloudy)
finely pared zest of 2 oranges
finely pared zest of 1 lemon
finely pared zest of 1 lime
1 cinnamon stick (about
   4cm/1½in, preferably Ceylon
   cinnamon)
1 piece of bitter orange peel
1½ tsp whole coriander seeds
½ star anise
½ tbsp finely grated fresh
   ginger root
2 green cardamom pods
4 dates
2 tbsp dried tamarind, peeled
   and finely chopped
2 whole mace
1 pinch of finely grated nutmeg
½ vanilla pod
1 tsp citric acid
½ tbsp salt

STEP 2
150g/5½oz/scant 1 cup dark
   muscovado sugar
100ml/3½fl oz/scant ⅔ cup dark
   syrup
400g/14oz/2 cups Demerara sugar
3 tbsp freshly squeezed orange
   juice (about 1 orange)
150ml/¼ pint/scant ⅔ cup freshly
   squeezed lemon juice (about
   2–3 lemons)

Bring all the ingredients from step 1 to the boil and leave to simmer for 30 minutes.

Remove from the heat and add all the ingredients from step 2, except the citrus. Leave to cool.

Add the citrus juices. Strain the mixture through a straining cloth or muslin and bottle in sterilised bottles.

Mix with carbonated water and ice.

CHERRY COLA

Mix half cola syrup with half of the syrup from Rob's Favourite Cherry Soda (page 37) together to make a Cherry Coke.

VANILLA COLA

Mix half Cola Syrup with half Cream Soda (page 24) together to make a Vanilla Coke. Squeeze in some extra lemon.

CRISPY ONION RINGS

When it comes to deep-frying, panko – Japanese breadcrumbs – are the star! You'll almost never fail when using panko – the result is always super crispy.

Serves 4
225g/8oz/1¾ cups plain flour
60g/2¼oz/1¼ cups panko
   breadcrumbs
2 eggs, beaten
1 litre/1¾ pints/4⅓ cups deep-
   frying oil, such as rapeseed
4 onions, sliced and separated
   into rings
salt flakes

Put the flour in two separate bowls. Put the panko in a third bowl and the eggs in a fourth. Heat the oil to 180°C/350°F.

Turn the onion rings in flour first, then dip them in beaten egg, once more in flour and one last time in the egg, then finally turn them over in panko.

Fry until golden brown, about 1–2 minutes. Leave to drain on a piece of kitchen paper, then sprinkle with salt.

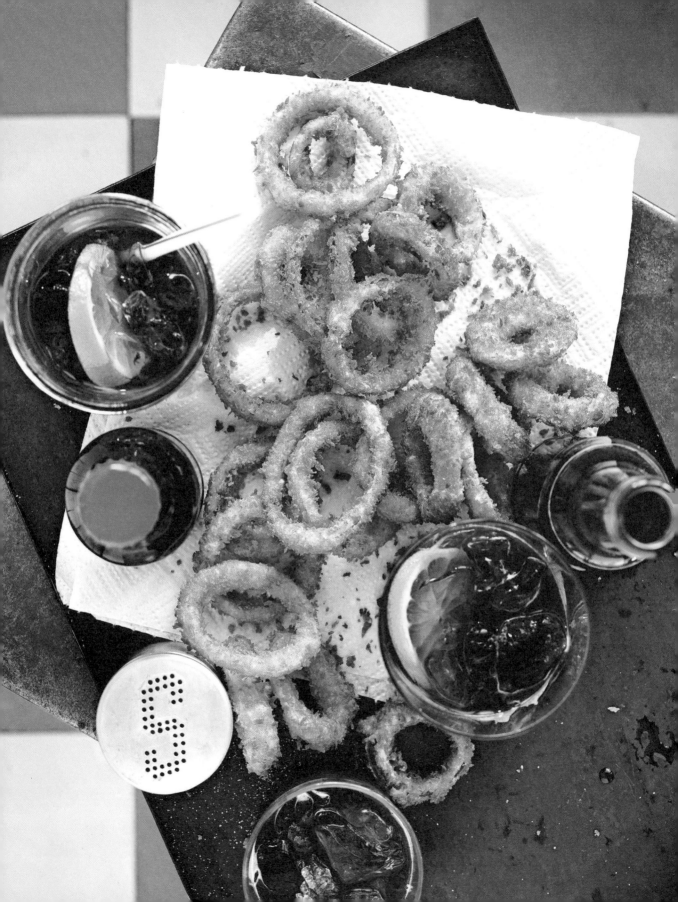

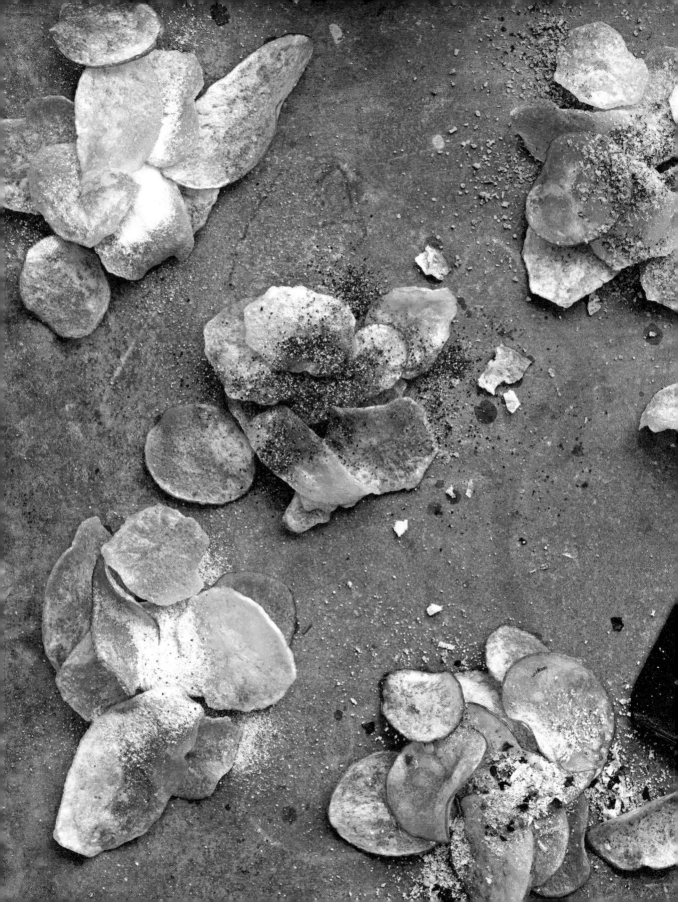

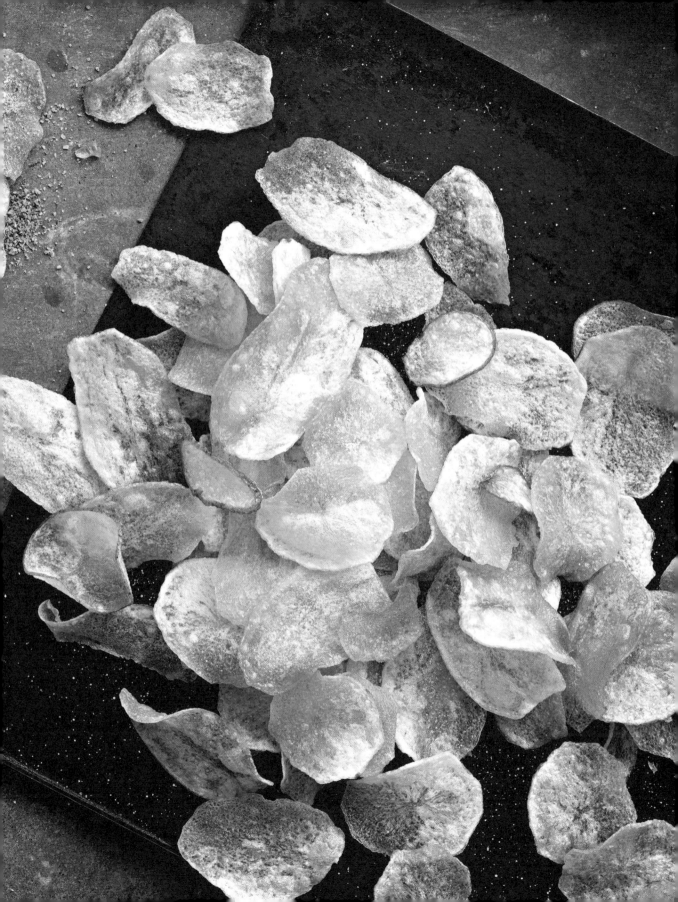

CHIPS *and* DIPS

Frying your own crisps gives super-tasty results. Plus, it feels a bit better to see oil bubbling around a locally grown potato rather than throwing a big bag of crisps into your shopping basket.

CRISPS

To achieve perfectly crispy crisps you should choose a firm potato variety, preferably use a deep-fryer that maintains exactly 150°C/300°F during the whole frying process and use a mandolin to get really even, thin slices of potato.

4–8 snack portions
8 firm potatoes
1.5 litres/2½ pints/6½ cups deep-frying oil, such as rapeseed
salt

Keep the peel on the potatoes or peel it off. It the potato is peeled it has to go straight into cold water so it doesn't get discoloured.

Slice the potatoes thinly using a mandolin, about 1–2mm/¹⁄₁₆in. If the slices get too thick they won't go crispy, and if they're too thin they will burn and taste more of oil than of potato.

Heat the oil to 150°C/350°F. Deep-fry the potato slices in batches for about 2 minutes, until they've coloured and have turned crisp. Stir the oil occasionally during frying so that the potato slices don't stick together. Take the potato slices out of the oil and leave to drain on kitchen paper.

Toss the crisps with salt or flavouring of your choice while still a little warm.

FLAVOURED CRISPS

Flavour the crisps when they're newly fried. Toss a batch of crisps in a large bowl together with about 1½ tsp flavoured salt. The spice mixes are also nice to mix with freshly popped popcorn.

SMOKY PAPRIKA CRISPS
1 tsp smoked paprika powder
2 pinches of ground chipotle chilli
1 tsp onion powder
1 tbsp salt

Mix all the ingredients together in a pestle and mortar so they are crushed into a powder. Toss with a batch of freshly fried crisps.

DILL & ONION CRISPS
1½ tbsp salt
3 tbsp finely chopped dill
½ tsp onion powder

Preheat the oven to 70°C/150°F (preferably a fan assisted oven). Blend the salt and dill in a food processor until the salt has become green and the dill is finely chopped. Place on an oven tray lined with baking parchment. Dry in the centre of the oven for about 20 minutes.

Take out and leave to cool and dry for a little longer at room temperature. Mix with the onion powder and crush into a fine powder using a pestle and mortar. Toss with a batch of freshly fried crisps.

CORIANDER, CHILLI & LIME CRISPS
1½ tbsp salt
4 tbsp finely chopped coriander
finely grated zest of 2 limes
1 tsp cumin
½ tsp chilli flakes

Preheat the oven to 70°C/150°F and line a baking tray with baking parchment. Blend the salt, coriander, lime zest, cumin and chilli flakes in a food processor until finely chopped. Bake for about 20 minutes.

Take out and leave to cool and dry at room temperature. Crush in a pestle and mortar until the lime zest is powdered. Toss with a batch of freshly fried crisps.

TRUFFLE & CHANTERELLE CRISPS
3–4 tbsp dried chanterelles
1½ tbsp salt
½ tsp white truffle oil

Blend the chanterelles and salt in a food processor. Crush into a powder using a pestle and mortar, then sift through a fine sieve. Mix with a batch of freshly fried crisps and the truffle oil.

SALT & VINEGAR CRISPS
2 tbsp salt
2 tbsp white wine vinegar
1½ tsp tartaric acid

Before you make the crisps, soak the potato slices in 200ml/7fl oz/scant 1 cup white wine vinegar about 1½ hours

You'll find recipes for dips on the next spread ... ➡

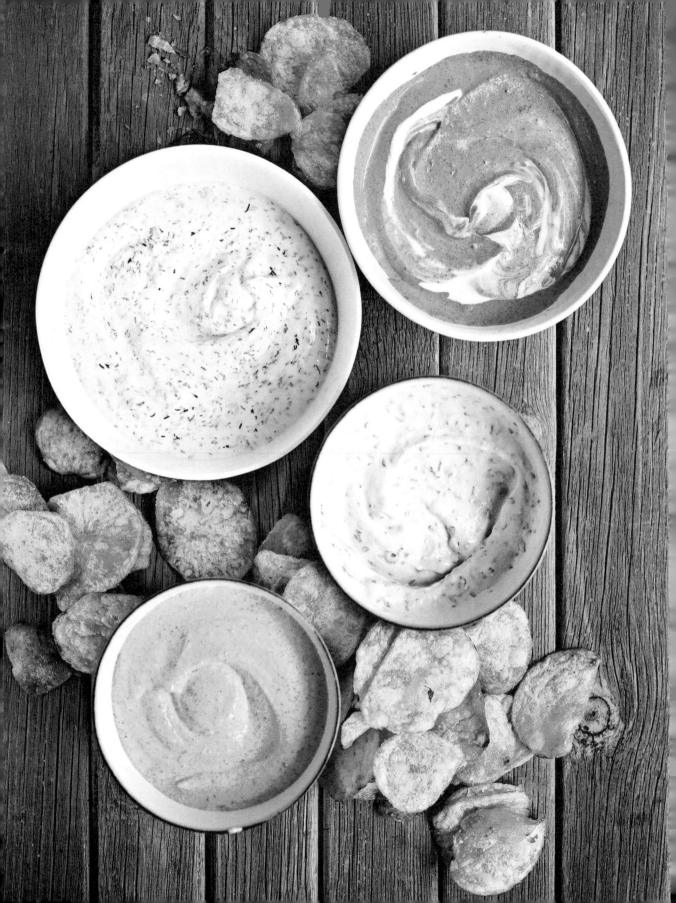

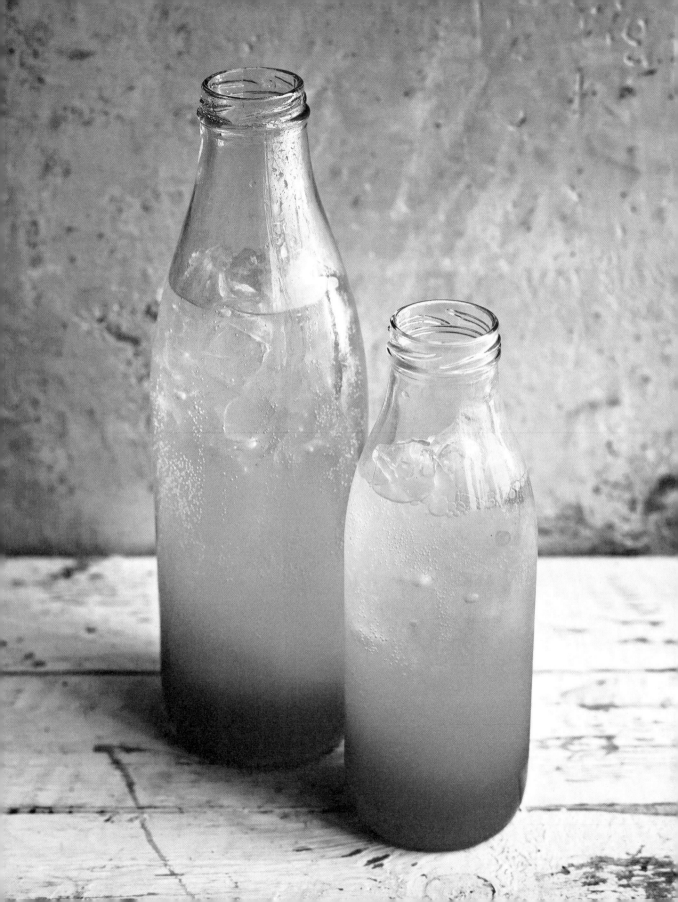

before frying. Take out and drain on a clean tea towel. Preheat the oven to 70°C/150°F.

Mix the salt, vinegar and tartaric acid in a small bowl. Pour onto an oven tray lined with baking parchment. Dry in the centre of the oven for about 1 hour, stirring occasionally.

Crush into a powder using a pestle and mortar. Toss with a batch of freshly fried crisps.

DIPS

A dip should be thick and creamy with a lot of flavour so that it's enough to dip only once. Ready-made dips often contain a thickening agent or stabiliser to make it thick and creamy, but I use soured cream and quark. Leave the dip to stand for at least 15 minutes in the fridge to develop the flavours before it's served.

4–8 snack portions

HOT PAPRIKA
240ml/8fl oz/1 cup soured cream, 240fl oz/8fl oz/1 cup cottage cheese, 1 tsp smoked paprika, 2 pinches of chilli flakes, 1 tsp onion powder and ½ tsp salt.

DILL & ONION
240ml/8fl oz/1 cup soured cream, 240ml/8fl oz/1 cup quark, 1 tsp dried dill, 1 tsp onion powder and ½ tsp salt.

TACO
240ml/8fl oz/1 cup soured cream, 240ml/8fl oz/1 cup quark, 1 tsp ground smoked paprika, ½ tsp cumin, ½ tsp onion powder and ½ tsp salt.

SOURED CREAM & ONION
240ml/8fl oz/1 cup soured cream, 240ml/8fl oz/1 cup quark, 1 tsp chopped parsley, 1 tsp onion powder, 1½ pinches of citric acid and ½ tsp salt.

CURRY
240ml/8fl oz/1 cup soured cream, 240ml/8fl oz/1 cup quark, 1 tsp curry powder, ½ tsp garam masala, ½ tsp onion powder and ½ tsp salt.

SEA BUCKTHORN TROCADERO

Trocadero is a classic Swedish drink that always springs to mind when I get a whiff of the fantastic tropical-fruit scent of these yellow sea-buckthorn berries. They are quite similar to passion fruit both in flavour and colour.

The berries are boiled with apple juice and citric acid so the result is fresh and sharp.

About 400ml/14fl oz/1¾ cups
200g/7oz/heaped 1 cup granulated sugar
200ml/7fl oz/scant 1 cup apple juice (clear not cloudy)
200ml/7fl oz/scant 1 cup water
100g/3½oz sea buckthorn berries
1 tsp citric acid

Melt 150g/5½oz/¾ cup sugar in a pan until golden brown. Remove from the heat.

Add the apple juice and water, being careful as the heat from the sugar might splash. The sugar will set and line the bottom like a lid. Lift the sugar carefully with a fork or a spoon so that it dissolves in the liquid. Add the remaining sugar, the sea buckthorn and citric acid. Leave to simmer gently without a lid for 15 minutes.

Sieve through a straining cloth or muslin and pour into a sterilised bottle. Leave to cool and store in the fridge.

LINGONBERRY & ANISEED SYRUP

This is made from coconut sugar, making it slightly less sweet. The soda will have a dry character with a liquorice tone from the star anise.

About 400ml/14fl oz/1¾ cups
225g/8oz/1¾ cups lingonberries
200ml/7fl oz/scant 1 cup coconut sugar
1 star anise
1 pinch of dried thyme
400ml/14fl oz/1¾ cups water

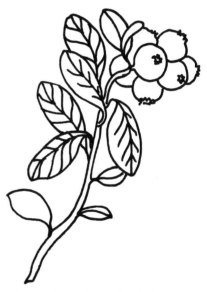

Bring all the ingredients to the boil in a pan, then simmer gently for about 30 minutes.

Run through a fine sieve, then pour into a sterilised jar. Cool, then store in the fridge.

CARBONATED *infusions*

The word infusion sounds a bit tricky, but don't let that put you off. An infusion is simply a liquid with a concentrated flavour from, for example, herbs and roots. Such concoctions have been used through the ages as calming drinks and to cure illnesses. In recent years, infusions have started to pop up on the menus of finer restaurants as an alternative to wine or beer. Seasonal herbs, roots and leaves are gathered and combined to find flavours that match with the food.

To make an infusion you pour warm water over a good bunch of herbs or roots and leave it to steep until the liquid has soaked up a lot of flavour. The liquid can then be mixed together with sparkling or still water and ice. I like to mix it with freshly squeezed juice for extra freshness and because juice goes very well with a sparkling infusion. Infusions that aren't sweetened are very nice to serve at meal times as the herby flavour often marries well with any herbiness in the food. Consider this: a fillet of fish or a rib eye steak that's fried with butter and herbs, perhaps some garlic, and then served with a glass of ice-cold bubbling water flavoured with thyme, rosemary and mild citrus – it doesn't get any better!

Here it's really possible to create your own recipes. Pick whatever you can find in the garden, in pots on the balcony, in the woods or hedgerow. Flowers, leaves, herbs, roots, citrus – all can be mixed into tasty and refreshing drinks.

BASIC INFUSION

Bring 400ml / 14fl oz / 1¾ cups of water to the boil, remove from the heat and leave to stand for 1 minute. Pour the hot water over one of the herb mixes below, or over other ingredients of your choice. Leave to stand until the water is cool. Add about 100ml / 3½fl oz / scant ½ cup freshly squeezed lemon or lime juice. Strain through a fine sieve. Store in a cool place.

> Allow for about 3–4 tbsp infusion to 200ml/7fl oz/scant 1 cup sparkling water.

HERB & LEMON

Infusion made from sage, rosemary and thyme with fresh notes of lemon.

400ml/14fl oz/1¾ cups water
25g/1oz/½ cup freshly picked thyme leaves
25g/1oz/½ cup freshly picked rosemary leaves
25g/1oz/½ cup freshly picked sage leaves
zest of 1 lemon

GINGER, DANDELION & MINT

Dandelion root has long been used in the production of naturally fermented drinks, just like ginger. The flavour becomes flowery and herby. With the addition of ginger and mint, this drink is really refreshing in an ice-filled glass with a slice of lemon.

400ml/14fl oz/1¾ cups water
60g/2¼oz/½ cup finely chopped fresh root ginger
10 dandelion flower heads
25g/1oz/½ cup freshly picked mint leaves
¼ vanilla pod and seeds, split lengthways

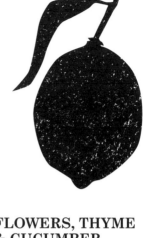

FLOWERS, THYME & CUCUMBER

Flowery infusion made from lavender, rosebuds and thyme.

400ml/14fl oz/1¾ cups water
25g/1oz/½ cup dried lavender
2 tbsp dried rosebuds
25g/1oz/½ cup freshly picked thyme leaves
finely grated zest of 1 lime
½ cucumber, sliced

CITRUS & GINGER

Infusion with orange, grapefruit, lemon, bitter lemon and ginger. Peel the citrus fruits with a knife, but avoid the white part, which can give a bitter flavour. Although, if it's the bitter notes that you are after, try instead to include as much white as possible.

400ml/14fl oz/1¾ cups water
zest of 2 oranges
zest of 2 grapefruits
zest of 1 lemon
2 dried bitter lemon peel
100g/3½oz finely chopped fresh root ginger

LEMONADE
and
ICED TEA

It's hard to beat a really ice-cold lemonade or iced tea on a hot summer's day. It's easy to think that there aren't that many variations of lemonade, but there are actually an infinite number of them – almost too many to choose from.

The base is citrus, water and sugar or other sweetener, such as honey or syrup. Unlike soda, a classic lemonade isn't carbonated but is more similar to a refreshing citrus-fresh cordial. You can make it fizzy by adding sparkling water instead of still. It's also often cold-mixed and considerably sharper than the sweet cordial. In the lemonade family you can also include the Mexican refreshing drink agua fresca – made from fresh fruit and a dash of citrus. Truly summer in a glass!

To serve your guests homemade lemonade is always a cheerful experience – everyone will be amazed that you've made your own and will gulp down the ice-cold drink in no time. Many people think it's difficult, but it's one of the simplest things you can do. How hard is it to squeeze a lemon and mix the juice with sugar and water? Not at all!

I would actually go so far as to say that a life without lemonade is an awful lot more boring. As the old saying goes: 'If life gives you lemons, make lemonade' – yes, lemonade will simply cheer you up.

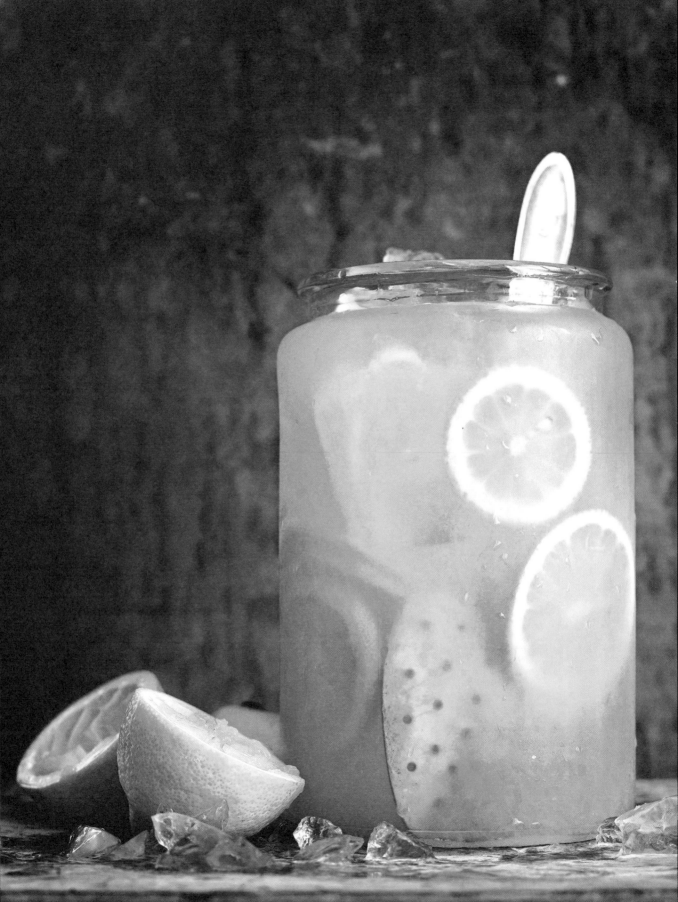

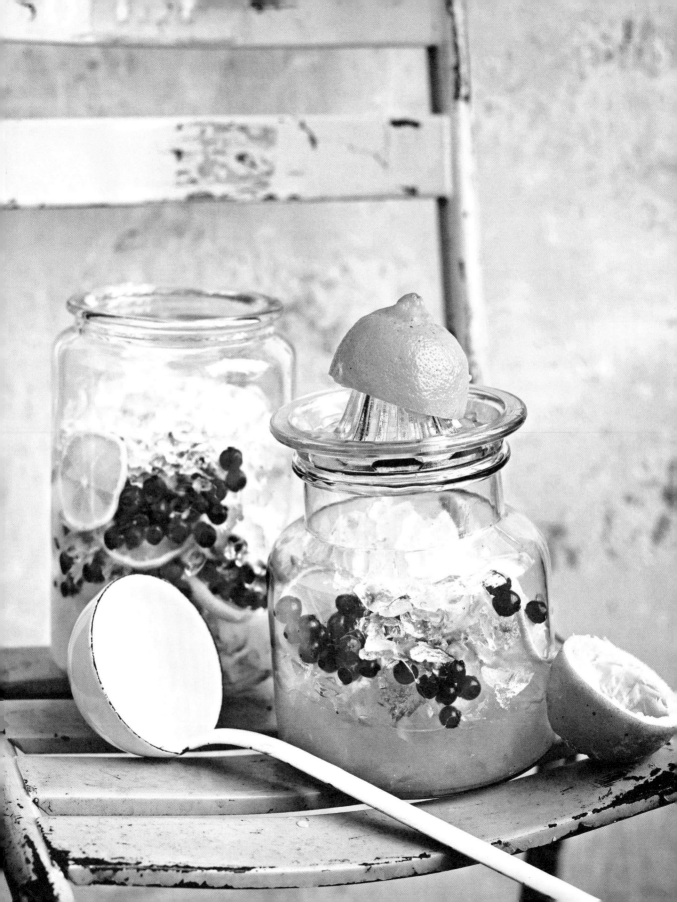

RED CURRANT LEMONADE

Red currants, raspberries, blackberries, blueberries, cloudberries, strawberries… It's great to muddle any of these into this type of lemonade. When you muddle the berries, instead of blending them, the whole berry is still left to give a fresh flavour and good texture – from stones to pulp.

About 1 litre/1¾ pints/4 ⅓ cups
225g/8oz/1½ cups granulated
   sugar
1 litre/1¾ pints/4⅓ cups water
crushed ice
150g/5½oz/1½ cups red currants
200ml/7fl oz/scant 1 cup freshly
   squeezed lemon juice
   (about 3-4 lemons)

Dissolve the sugar in 100ml/3½fl oz/scant ½ cup of the water in a pan over a low heat. Leave to cool.

Fill a large jug half full of crushed ice. Add the currants, syrup and freshly squeezed lemon juice. Crush with a ladle or a muddler. Add the remaining water and serve immediately.

CLASSIC LEMONADE

Lemonade can be boiled like a cordial or mixed cold. On a hot summer's day when you want a refreshing glass of lemonade really quickly, it's all about the classic version. It's cold-mixed and gets a nice freshness from the freshly squeezed lemons, sugar and ice. For a more concentrated lemonade you use less water and vice versa for a less concentrated lemonade.

About 1.5 litres/2½ pints/6½ cups
100g/3½oz/½ cup granulated sugar
250ml/9fl oz/generous 1 cup
   freshly squeezed lemon juice
   (about 5 lemons)
1 litre/1¾ pints/4⅓ cups water

Mix the sugar with the lemon juice in a large jug (about 1.5 litre/2½ pint/6½ cup capacity). Leave to stand for about 10 minutes, stirring occasionally, until the sugar has dissolved.

Fill the jug with ice and add water. Stir into a cold lemonade. Dilute with more water, if needed, and check the taste. Some people like it intensely sweet-sharp and others like it a bit more diluted and refreshing. (See photograph on page 51.)

BARLEY WATER

This is a British classic, although making drinks from grains isn't unique to Britain. Traces have been found suggesting that the ancient Greeks drank a fresh drink made from grains in between their glasses of wine. In Mexico there's horchata made from rice grains; in Scotland Atholl brose, made from oats and whisky; and mugicha brewed from grains is common in Asia. In Great Britain it's all about barley water made from barley grains and lemons.

About 2.5 litres/4½ pints/
   2½ quarts
85g/3oz/scant ½ cup pearl barley
150ml/¼ pint/scant ⅔ cup
   + 1.5 litres/2½ pints/6½ cups
   water
finely grated zest of 5–6 lemons
200ml/7fl oz/scant 1 cup freshly
   squeezed lemon juice (about
   5–6 lemons)

Boil the pearl barley in 150ml/ ¼ pint/scant ⅔ cup of the water for about 30 minutes, adding a little extra water if necessary. Strain through a fine sieve and leave to cool.

Bring 1.5 litres/2½ pints/ 6½ cups water to the boil with the sugar. Remove from the heat and stir in the lemon zest. Leave to cool.

Mix the cool lemon liquid with lemon juice and barley liquid. Serve ice-cold.

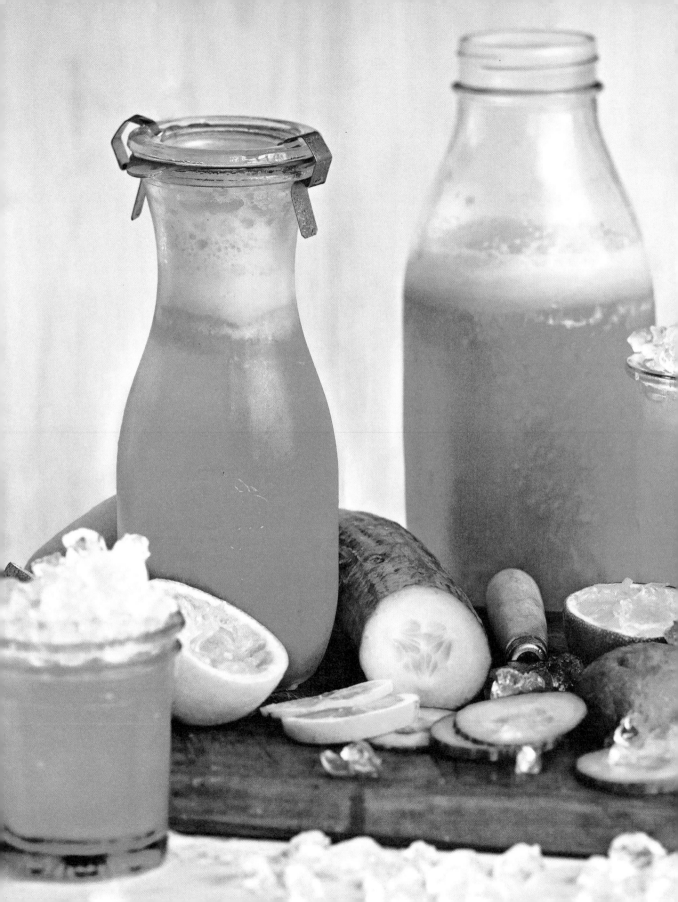

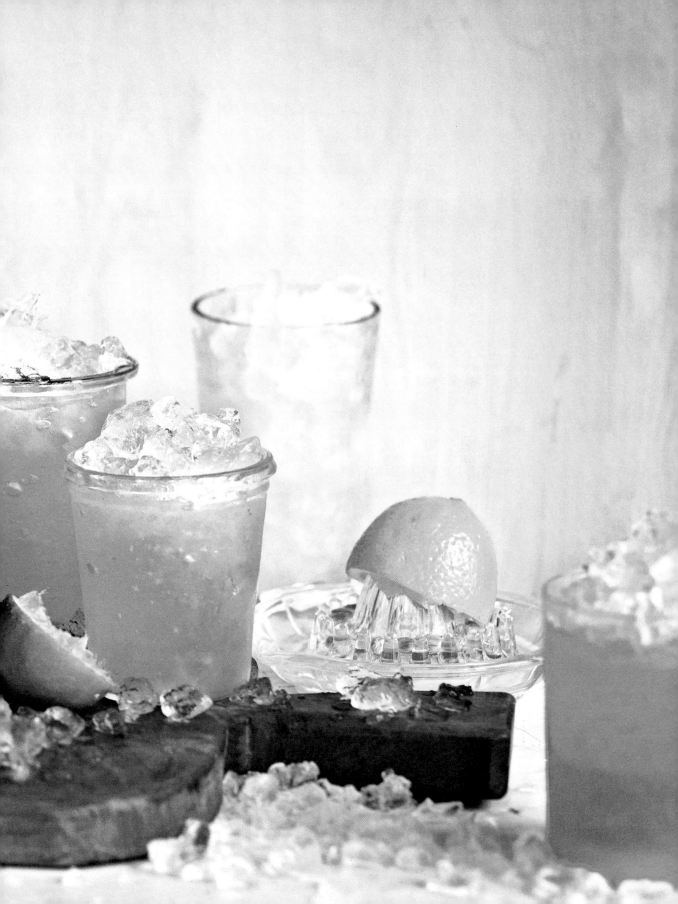

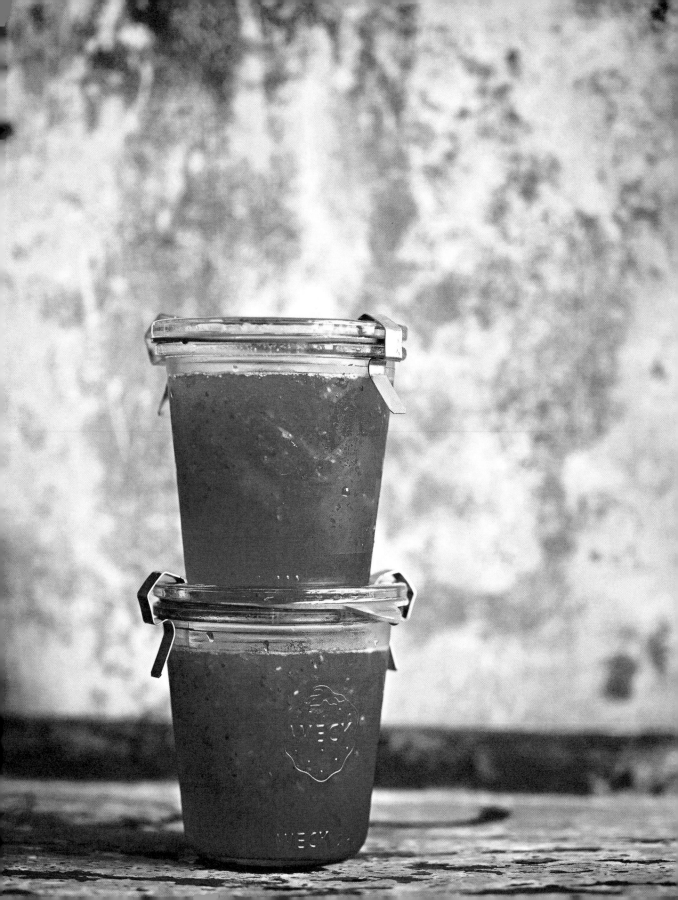

GREEN CUCUMBER LEMONADE

A properly fresh lemonade with a taste of cucumber that gives the ultimate coolness to quench your thirst.

About 1.5 litres/2½ pints/6½ cups
100ml/3½fl oz/scant ½ cup freshly
    squeezed lemon juice
    (about 1½–2 lemons)
100ml/3½fl oz/scant ½ cup freshly
    squeezed lime juice
    (about 3 limes)
1 cucumber, rinsed and diced
150ml/¼ pint/scant ⅔ cup clear
    honey
25g/1oz/½ cup chopped fresh mint
    leaves
25g/1oz/½ cup chopped fresh
    lemon balm leaves
1.2 litres/generous 2 pints/
    5 cups water

Mix together the citrus juice, cucumber, honey, mint, lemon balm and half the water in a blender. Blend thoroughly until the liquid is bright green and the mint, lemon balm and cucumber are puréed. Strain though a fine sieve.

Add the remaining water and adjust the flavour with more citrus and honey, if needed. Serve in glasses filled with ice. (See photograph on pages 54–55.)

RASPBERRY & CHIA LEMONADE

The Mexicans have been mixing drinks with chia seeds for a long time. This drink is jam-packed with omega-3 fatty acids, proteins, vitamins and minerals: a perfect lemonade to choose when you need extra power in the heat.

About 1.5 litres/2½ pints/6½ cups
1 litre/1¾ pints/4⅓ cups water
150g/5½oz/¾ cup Demerara sugar
200g/7oz/scant 1½ cups
    raspberries
3 tbsp chia seeds
250ml/9fl oz/generous 1 cup
    freshly squeezed lime juice
    (about 6–7 limes)

Mix together the water, sugar and raspberries using a blender. Strain through a fine sieve into a large jug.

Stir in the chia seeds and lime juice. Leave to stand for 10 minutes to let the chia seeds absorb the liquid. Stir and adjust the flavour with more sugar or lime, if needed. Serve with ice.

GRAPEFRUIT LEMONADE

About 1 litre/1¾ pints/4⅓ cups
4 grapefruits (pink if you like)
½ tsp citric acid
100g/3½oz/½ cup granulated sugar
700ml/24fl oz/3 cups water
3 tbsp freshly squeezed lemon
    juice (about 1 lemon)
1 pot of lemon balm

Peel 2 of the grapefruits with a knife or a vegetable peeler, and include the white part as it will give the lemonade a nice bitter character. Squeeze the juice from all 4 grapefruits. You should have about 400ml/14fl oz/1¾ cups.

Mix the grapefruit peel, citric acid, sugar and 300ml/½ pint/1¼ cups of the water in a pan. Bring to the boil, then remove from the heat. Add the remaining water, then leave the mixture to cool.

Run through a fine sieve, then add the grapefruit and lemon juice.

Mix together with a handful of lemon balm leaves in a jug and serve with ice.

SALTY LEMONADE

Salty lemonade is served in a lot of places around the world. It is perfect in hotter countries as you often get a craving for salt after a hot day in the sun.

About 1 litre/1¾ pints/4⅓ cups
100ml/3½fl oz/scant ½ cup freshly squeezed lemon juice (about 1½–2 lemons)
100ml/3½fl oz/scant ½ cup freshly squeezed grapefruit juice (about 1 grapefruit)
100ml/3½fl oz/scant ½ cup freshly squeezed lime juice (about 3 limes)
225g/8oz/1½ cups granulated sugar, plus extra for the glasses
½ tsp salt, plus extra for the glasses
1 litre/1¾ pints/4⅓ cups water

Mix together the citrus juices with the sugar and salt. Leave to stand for about 15 minutes, stirring occasionally, until the sugar has dissolved.

Mix together equal parts of sugar and salt on a plate. Run a lime wedge along the edges of the glasses and dip them in the sugar mixture.

Fill the glasses with ice. Mix the citrus liquid with water and pour into the glasses.

NUTS FOR NUTS

Sweet-salty nuts with a spicy sting!

Serves 6–8
400g/4oz/3 cups nuts, for example almonds, hazelnuts or cashew nuts
3 tbsp clear honey
1 tsp salt flakes
1 tsp ground coriander
½ ground cumin
1 tsp ground ancho chillies, Spanish smoked ground paprika or ground chipotle chilli

Preheat the oven to 170°C/325°F/Gas 3 and line a baking tray with baking parchment. Mix together all the ingredients on the prepared tray.

Roast in the middle of the oven for about 15 minutes until the kitchen starts smelling of roasted nuts and the honey has caramelised around the nuts.

Tip the nuts onto baking parchment and leave to cool. Fill into paper cones and serve.

Tip!
Swap the honey for 1 egg white if you don't want the sweetness.

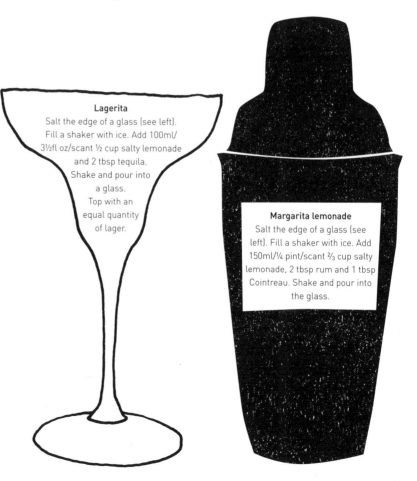

Lagerita
Salt the edge of a glass (see left). Fill a shaker with ice. Add 100ml/3½fl oz/scant ½ cup salty lemonade and 2 tbsp tequila. Shake and pour into a glass. Top with an equal quantity of lager.

Margarita lemonade
Salt the edge of a glass (see left). Fill a shaker with ice. Add 150ml/¼ pint/scant ⅔ cup salty lemonade, 2 tbsp rum and 1 tbsp Cointreau. Shake and pour into the glass.

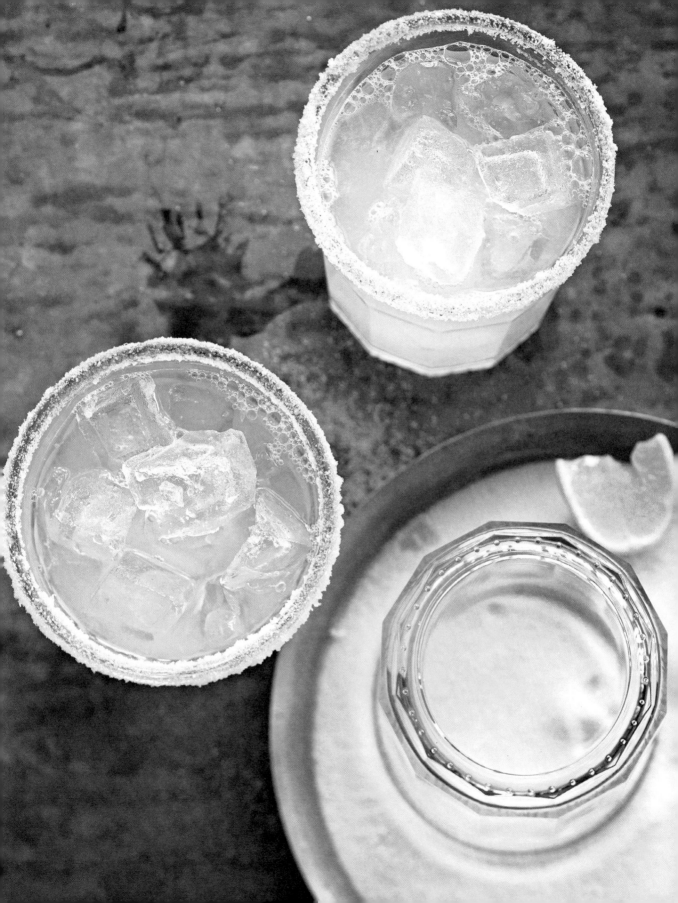

RHUBARB & BASIL LEMONADE

Sour and fresh rhubarb is nice with herby basil. The basil can be replaced with mint, thyme, rosemary or lemon balm.

About 1 litre/1¾ pints/4⅓ cups
200g/7oz rhubarb, sliced
100g/3½oz/½ cup granulated sugar
600ml/1 pint/1¼ cups water
3 tbsp freshly squeezed lime juice and finely grated zest (about 2 limes)
500ml/17fl oz/generous 2 cups water
100ml/3½fl oz/scant ½ cup freshly squeezed lemon juice (about 1½–2 lemons)
a few basil leaves

Bring the rhubarb, sugar and 600ml/1 pint/1¼ cups water to the boil and simmer for about 5 minutes. Remove from the heat and add the lime juice and zest and remaining water. Leave to cool.

Run through a fine sieve, then mix with the lemon juice. Serve in ice-filled glasses together with a few basil leaves.

ELDERFLOWER & STRAWBERRY LEMONADE

About 1.5 litres/2½ pints/6½ cups
100ml/3½fl oz/scant ½ cup elderflower cordial
1 litre/1¾ pints/4⅓ cups water
150ml/¼ pint/scant ⅔ cup freshly squeezed lime juice (about 4–5 limes)
450g/1lb strawberries
few sprigs of mint

Blend together the elderflower cordial, water, lime juice and half of the strawberries using a stick blender.

Strain through a fine sieve. Slice the rest of the strawberries and mix together with ice and the blended liquid in a jug. Serve with mint in the glasses.

QUEEN LEMONADE

About 1 litre/1¾ pints/4⅓ cups
100g/3½oz raspberries
100g/3½oz blueberries
150g/5½oz/¾ cup Demerara sugar
150ml/¼ pint/scant ⅔ cup freshly squeezed lime juice (about 4–5 limes)
1 litre/1¾ pints/4⅓ cups water

Warm up half of the berries in a pan with the sugar and let the sugar dissolve. Remove from the heat and leave to cool.

Mix together with the lime juice and water, then strain through a fine sieve.

Add the rest of the berries and stir. Serve with ice.

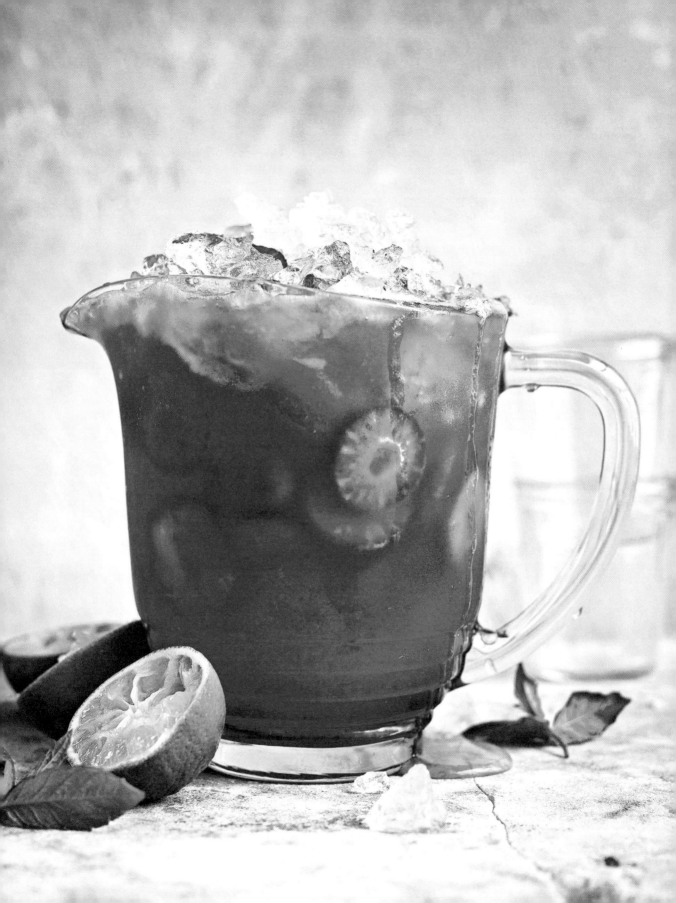

AGUA FRESCA

The Mexicans know how to make the most from tasty sun-ripened fruit and transform it into cooling drinks. Water and fruit is all that's needed. Along roadsides, at beaches, in town squares and cafés you find large jars and jugs with colourful drinks. It feels like being a child in a sweet shop, to stand and choose between pink watermelon, orange, pale lemon, purple hibiscus, yellow pineapple and red strawberry. If the fruits aren't sun-ripened and picked directly from the trees and bushes, like in Mexico, but instead come from the food store around the corner, you might need to boost the flavour with a little sugar and freshly squeezed citrus juice.

AGUA DE PIÑA

About 1 litre/1¾ pints/4⅓ cups
1 pineapple (about 1kg/2lb 4oz), peeled and diced
3 tbsp freshly squeezed lemon juice (about 1 lemon)
2 tbsp granulated sugar
600ml/1 pint/generous 2½ cups water

Mix the pineapple into a smooth juice together with the lemon, sugar and water in a blender.
  Strain through a fine sieve. Check the flavour to see if you need more lemon or sugar. Serve with ice.

AGUA DE SANDÍA

This is the tastiest thing in the world. Ice-cold watermelon and a dash of lime.

About 1 litre/1¾ pints/4⅓ cups
1 watermelon (about 2kg/4lb 8oz), peeled and diced
50g/1¾oz/¼ cup granulated sugar
100ml/3½fl oz/scant ½ cup freshly squeezed lime juice (about 3 limes)

Mix the melon, sugar and lime juice together in a blender. Run through a fine sieve. Serve with plenty of ice.

AGUA FRESCA DE TAMARINDO

A taste of dates and dried fruit but with a clear acidity – that's tamarind. The brown seed capsule with sticky fleshy seeds can be found in Asian food stores and good supermarkets. The sweet fruit with acidity breaking through is a perfect ingredient for cooling drinks.

About 1 litre/1¾ pints/4⅓ cups
1 litre/1¾ pints/4⅓ cups water
150g/5½oz tamarind
100g/3½oz/½ cup granulated sugar
2 tbsp freshly squeezed lime juice (about ½ lime)

Bring the water and tamarind to the boil in a large pan. Leave to simmer for about 30 minutes until the flesh falls off the stones. Strain through a fine sieve.
  Mix together with sugar and lime juice. Leave to cool. Serve in glasses filled with ice.

CANTALOUPE AGUA FRESCA

The key here is to find a ripe melon when it's in season, since the drink otherwise will taste quite dull. Sniff the melon – if it smells ripe, fruity and melony and feels a bit soft and juicy, then you can go ahead and mix a glass of cooling melon water.

About 1 litre/1¾ pints/4⅓ cups
1 cantaloupe melon (about 800g/1lb 12oz), peeled, seeds removed and flesh diced
2–3 tbsp granulated sugar
3 tbsp freshly squeezed lime juice (about 1–2 limes)
500ml/17fl oz/generous 2 cups water

Mix the melon, sugar, lime juice and water together in a blender. Run through a fine sieve. Serve with ice.

AGUA DE MANGO

Here it's all about ripe mango. The Thai or Pakistani ones with yellow skin have the best flavour and softest flesh.

About 1 litre/1¾ pints/4⅓ cups
400g/14oz mango, peeled and diced
3 tbsp granulated sugar
3 tbsp freshly squeezed lime juice (about 1–2 limes)
600ml/1 pint/generous 2½ cups ice-cold water

Blend the mango with sugar, lime juice and water into a smooth juice. Strain through a fine sieve. Check the flavour to see if you need to add more lime or sugar.

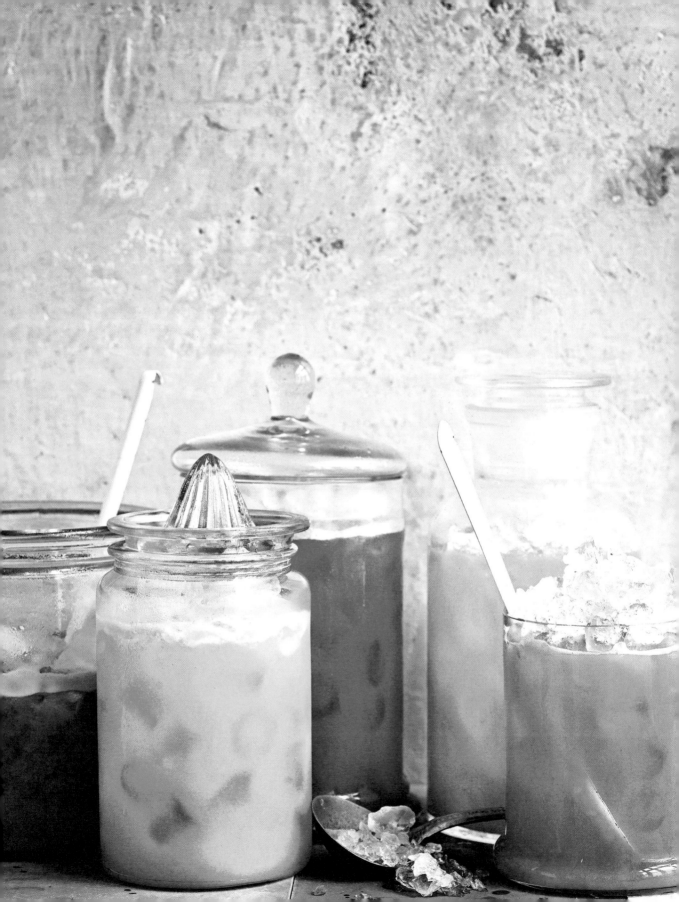

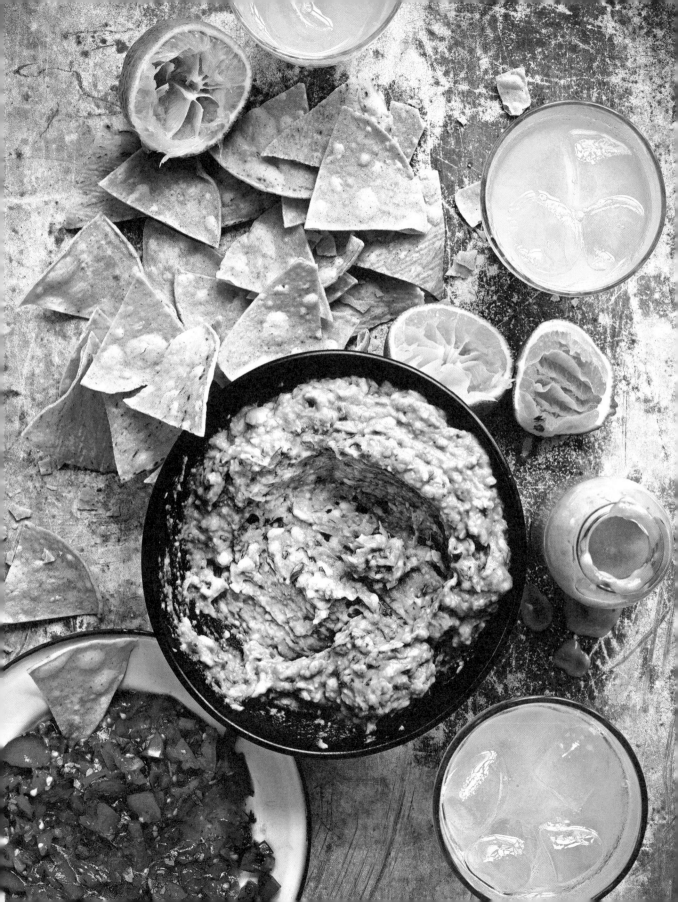

CRISPY CORN TORTILLAS

To make your own corn tortillas, you'll need a tortilla press to make them really thin. To succeed, you also have to use Latin American cornflour (masa harina), as cornmeal won't work very well for tortillas. If you can't make your own tortillas you can buy Mexican corn tortillas from major suppermarkets, Latin American shops or online. It will be thousand times nicer to deep-fry them yourself than to buy the ready-made crisps that are sold in food stores.

Makes about 15
300ml/½ pint/1¼ cups warm water
250g/9oz/2½ cups masa harina
a pinch of salt
1.5 litres/2½ pints/6½ cups deep-frying oil, such as rapeseed oil
salt flakes

Bring the water to the boil, pour into a bowl, then whisk in the cornflour. Add the salt and work into a springy dough. Divide the dough into 15 pieces and roll into balls. Press out in between two sheets of clingfilm in a tortilla press.

Heat a frying pan and fry the tortilla for about 1 minute on each side. They should bubble up and get a nice golden brown colour. Make sure the pan isn't too hot, or the tortilla will be more burnt than soft and nice.

Heat the oil to 170°C/325°F in a deep-fryer or a large pan. Slice the bread into wedges and fry until crispy for about 1 minute. Leave to drain on a piece of kitchen paper, then sprinkle with salt flakes.

SALSA FRESCA

A good salsa to serve with the tortilla crisps, this can be mixed with guacamole for variation.

4–6 portions
4 tomatoes, finely chopped
1 red chilli, deseeded and finely chopped
4 tbsp chopped fresh coriander
2 tbsp freshly squeezed lime juice (about 1 lime)
salt

Mix together the tomatoes, chilli, coriander and lime juice. Season with salt to taste.

GUACAMOLE

I don't use tomato in this guacamole. Instead you can serve it on the side in the form of salsa fresca.

4–6 portions
2 avocados
1 garlic clove, finely grated
1 jalapeño, deseeded and finely chopped
4 tbsp chopped fresh coriander
1 tbsp freshly squeezed lime juice (about ½ lime)
salt

Remove the stone from the avocados and mash up the flesh using a fork or a large pestle and mortar. Add the garlic, jalapeño and coriander. Season with lime juice and salt to taste.

SALSA AMARILLO

4–6 portions
3 yellow tomatoes, deseeded and cut into wedges
1 garlic clove, finely grated
2 yellow chillies, deseeded
1 tbsp freshly squeezed lime juice (about ½ lime)
salt

Mix the tomatoes with the rest of the ingredients using a stick blender, seasoning with lime juice and salt to taste.

SALSA ROJA

4–6 portions
3 red tomatoes, deseeded and cut into wedges
1 garlic clove, finely grated
2 red chillies, deseeded
1 tbsp freshly squeezed lime juice (about ½ lime)
salt

Mix the tomatoes together with the rest of the ingredients using a stick blender, seasoning with lime juice and salt to taste.

SALSA VERDE

4–6 portions
3 green or yellow tomatoes, deseeded and cut into wedges
1 garlic clove, finely grated
4 tbsp finely chopped fresh coriander
1 tbsp freshly squeezed lime juice (about ½ lime)
salt

Mix the tomatoes with the rest of the ingredients using a stick blender, seasoning with lime juice and salt to taste.

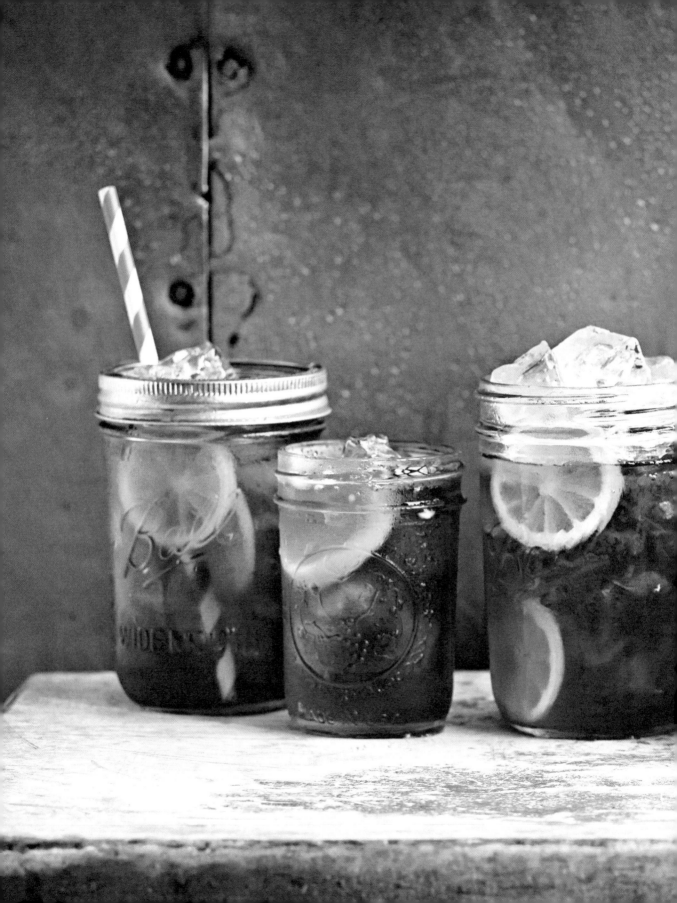

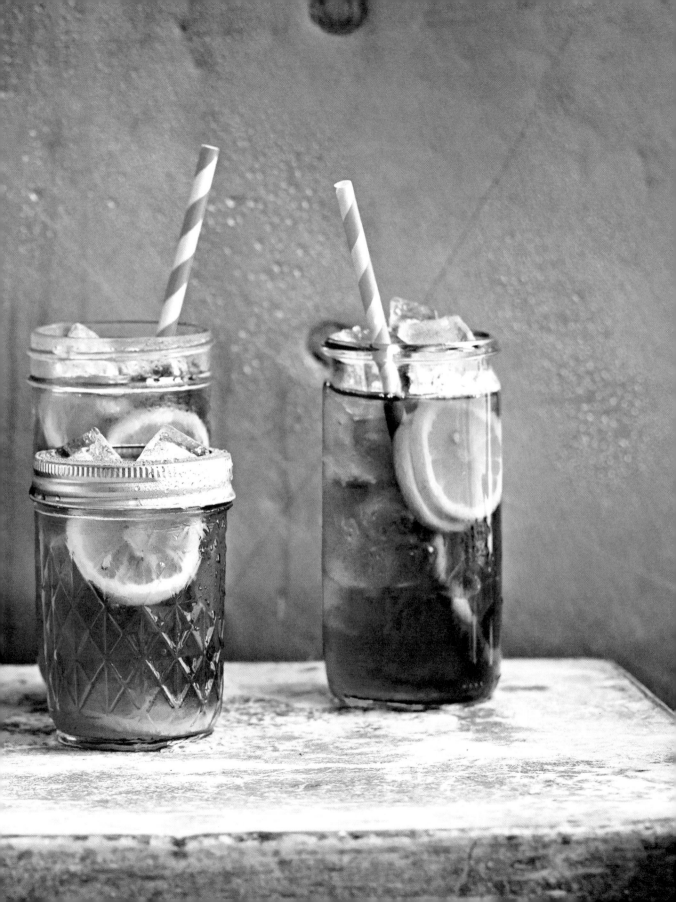

ICED TEAS

In the summer I always have a jug of iced tea in the fridge. The perfect thirst quencher, it can also be varied into infinity. Flavour it with different kinds of tea, fruit, berries and spices. (See photograph on pages 66–67.)

BASIC ICED TEA

About 1 litre/1¾ pints/4⅓ cups
1 litre/1¾ pints/4⅓ cups water
2 tbsp tea (black or green)
150g/5½oz/¾ cup Demerara sugar
3 tbsp freshly squeezed lemon
   juice (about 1 lemon)
lemon slices, to serve

Bring half the water to the boil in a pan. Add the tea and leave it to steep for about 5 minutes.

Strain and mix with the sugar. Leave to cool, stirring a few times so the sugar dissolves.

Mix with the remaining water and the lemon juice and place in the fridge. Serve with ice and a slice of lemon.

JASMINE & PEACH ICED TEA

This is a deluxe iced tea. You should preferably use the green jasmine tea, sencha, to make the drink perfect. The mildly perfumed flavour from the jasmine and the fruit of ripe peach will be a favourite in an ice-filled glass.

About 1 litre/1¾ pints/4⅓ cups
2 ripe peaches
1 litre/1¾ pints/4⅓ cups water
2 tbsp green jasmine tea (sencha)
50g/1¾oz/¼ cup Demerara sugar
3 tbsp freshly squeezed lemon
   juice (about 1 lemon)
lemon slices, to serve

Peel and cut the peaches into small pieces. Blend half into a smooth purée using a stick blender, then strain through a fine sieve.

Bring half the water to the boil in a pan. Add the tea and leave to steep for about 5 minutes. Strain and mix with the sugar and peach purée. Stir until the sugar has dissolved, then add the remaining water. Leave to cool.

Mix with the lemon juice and the reserved peach pieces and place in the fridge. Serve with ice and a slice of lemon.

CHAI ICED TEA

About 1 litre/1¾ pints/4⅓ cups
500ml/17fl oz/generous 2 cups
   water
3 tbsp clear honey
50g/1¾oz/¼ cup Demerara sugar
1 tbsp coarsely ground cardamom
   seeds
2 cinnamon sticks
1 tbsp black tea, preferably
   English breakfast, or flavoured
   with cinnamon or cardamom
500ml/17fl oz/generous 2 cups
   whole milk

Bring the water to the boil with honey, sugar, cardamom and three-quarters of the cinnamon. Remove from the heat and add the tea. Leave to cool. Add the milk and serve with ice.

MINTY ICED TEA

About 1 litre/1¾ pints/4⅓ cups
1 litre/1¾ pints/4⅓ cups water
2 tbsp black tea, preferably
   Earl Grey
50g/1¾oz/¼ cup Demerara sugar
25g/1oz/½ cup chopped fresh mint
3 tbsp freshly squeezed lime juice
   (about 1–2 limes)

Bring half the water to the boil. Add the tea and sugar, then leave to cool.

Add the remaining water and blend together with the mint using a stick blender or ordinary blender. Run through a fine sieve. Add the lime juice and serve with ice.

PINK LEMONADE

Light pink lemonade with a taste of pomegranate. Here you can vary the citrus fruits and use lime instead of lemon, or perhaps try half lemon and half grapefruit.

About 1 litre/1¾ pints/4⅓ cups
1 pomegranate
225g/8oz/1½ cups granulated sugar
250ml/9fl oz/generous 1 cup freshly squeezed lemon juice (about 5–6 lemons)
1.2 litres/generous 2 pints/5 cups water

Deseed the pomegranate and mix with the sugar and lemon juice in a bowl. Stir with a large spoon and press the pomegranate seeds towards the bowl so that the juice is squeezed out.

Strain and pour into a large jug or jar. Leave to stand for about 10 minutes, stirring occasionally until the sugar has dissolved.

Fill the jug with ice and add water. Stir into a cold lemonade. Dilute with more water, if needed. (See photograph on page 70.)

LOVELY ROSE LEMONADE

Citrus lemonade with a hint of rose petals. You can find rose water in large supermarkets or stores specialising in food from the Middle East.

About 1 litre/1¾ pints/4⅓ cups
150ml/¼ pint/scant ⅔ cup freshly squeezed lemon juice (about 2–3 lemons)
100g/3½oz/½ cup granulated sugar
1 small beetroot
2 splashes of rose water
1 litre/1¾ pints/4⅓ cups water

Mix the lemon juice and sugar in a bowl. Peel and coarsely grate the beetroot and stir into the lemon and sugar mixture. Leave to stand for about 30 minutes until the sugar has dissolved and the liquid has become red. Mix with the rose water and water.

Strain through a fine sieve into a jug and serve in ice-filled glasses. (See photograph on page 71.)

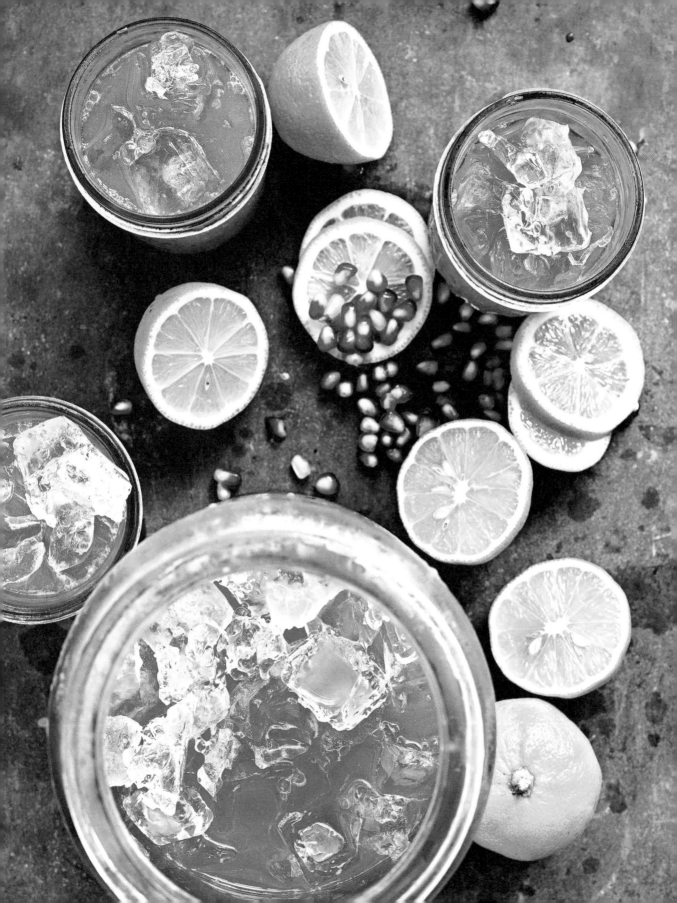

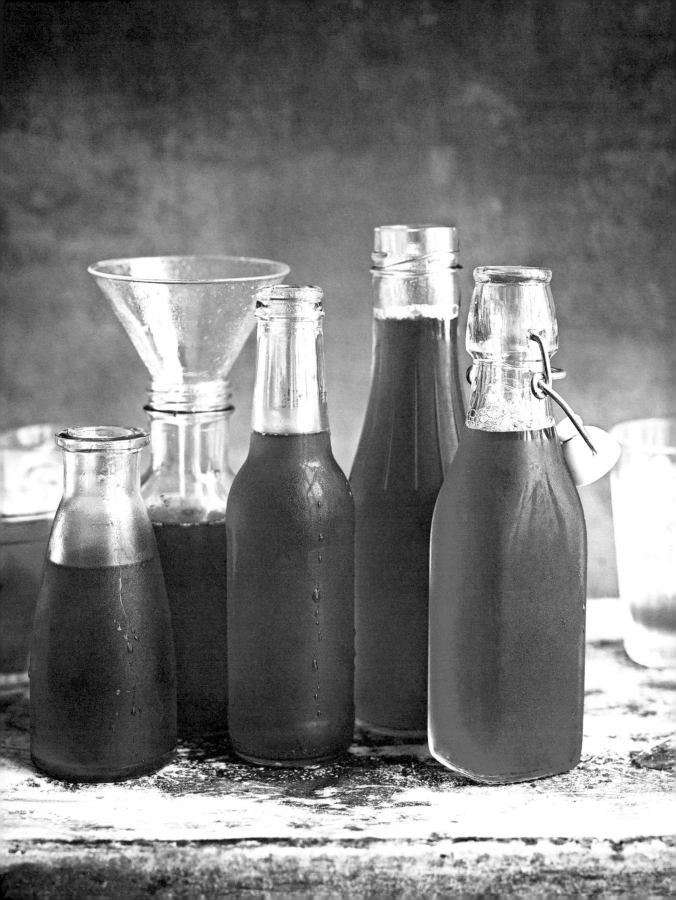

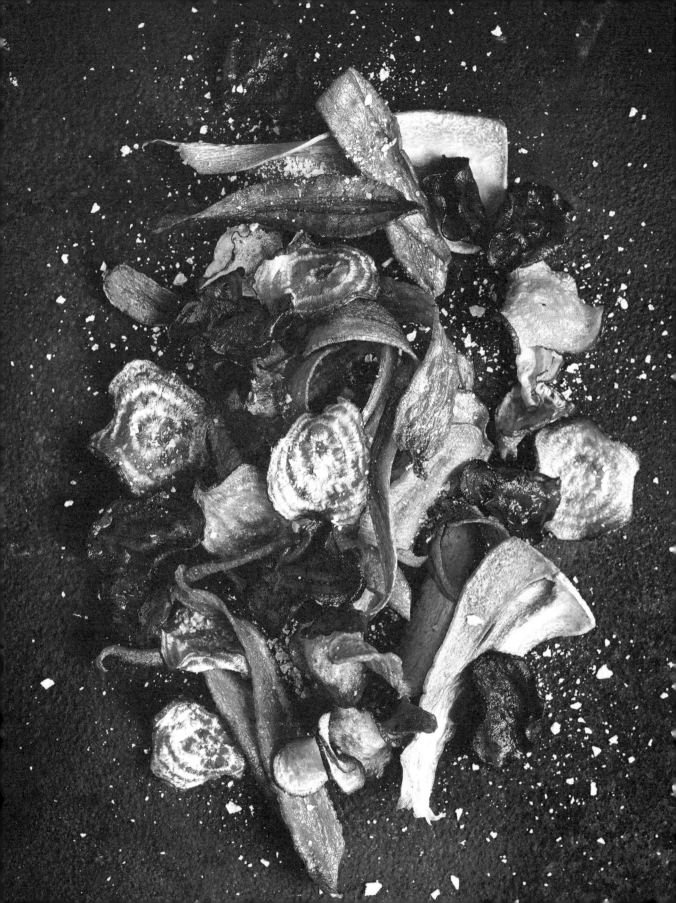

ROOT VEGETABLE CRISPS

Go ahead and choose whichever root veg you fancy. Both carrot and beetroot come in different colours and varieties and will look beautiful when deep-fried. A bowl full of deep-fried root vegetables and some salt flakes is a nice snack and the flavours truly come out when heated.

Serves 6–8
500g/1lb 2oz root vegetables, such as red and yellow beetroot, carrot, parsnip, sweet potato
about 1 litre/1¾ pints/4⅓ cups deep-frying oil, such as rapeseed
salt flakes

Rinse the root vegetables and dry them thoroughly. Slice thinly using a mandolin or a vegetable peeler.

Heat the oil to 150°C/300°F in a deep-fryer or a large pan. Deep-fry the root vegetables in batches. Start with the ones with the lightest colours and finish off with the darker ones, such as red beetroot, which will discolour the oil.

Deep-fry the vegetables until golden brown and crisp. Leave to drain on kitchen paper. Salt while they're still warm.

Leave to cool and store in an airtight jar for up to 2 weeks.

CHEESY KALE CHIPS

Probably one of the healthier snacks, kale is most often associated with being creamed, or in soup made from the Christmas leftovers, but the tasty green leaves can be used for so many more things. In fact kale now seems to be having a moment in the limelight – in the US, it pops up in anything from fine dining dishes to crisps. When the the kale hype has settled, these crisps will remain on the snack table, guaranteed. Crispy, cheesy, smoky and salty – way too delicious to be forgotten.

Serves 6–8
400g/14oz kale or cavolo nero
120g/4¼oz/1 cup cashew nuts
3 tbsp Japanese soy sauce
2 tbsp water
2 tbsp olive oil
1½ tsp Spanish smoked paprika
400g/14oz Parmesan cheese, finely grated
½ garlic clove, finely grated

Preheat the oven to 100°C/200°F and line two baking sheets with baking parchment. Rinse the kale, dry with a clean kitchen towel and cut into large pieces. Blend the nuts, soy sauce, water, oil, paprika, Parmesan and garlic to a paste using a stick blender.

Mix the kale with the blended paste in a large bowl, making sure all the kale is covered in paste. Spread out on the prepared baking sheets and dry in the oven for 30 minutes, then turn the oven down to 70°C/150°F and leave for a further 3½ hours. Open the oven door a few times during the first hour to let the steam out and turn the trays half way through. Turn the heat off and leave to cool in the oven.

Store in an airtight bag or jar for up to 2 weeks.

WARM ARTICHOKE DIP

A proper cheesy dip, warm, melted, thready, creamy cheese with artichoke and lemon. This dip is always a success as a condiment or snack with crisps or well-toasted baguette slices. This recipe is passed around my group of friends and I am probably asked at least once a month how to do it.

Serves 6–8
390g/13oz tin artichoke hearts
juice and finely grated zest of ¼ lemon
125g/4½oz Gouda cheese or other good cheese for melting, coarsely grated
125g/4½oz mozzarella cheese, coarsely grated
50g/1¾oz Parmesan cheese, finely grated
100ml/3½fl oz/scant ½ cup mayonnaise
2 egg yolks
½ tbsp finely chopped thyme
½ tsp salt flakes
a small pinch of black pepper

Preheat the oven to 250°C/500°F. Drain and chop the artichokes and squeeze out the liquid. Mix with the lemon zest and juice, cheeses, mayonnaise, egg yolks and thyme. Season with salt and pepper. Scoop into 2 round oven dishes (about 15cm/6in in diameter).

Bake in the middle of the oven for about 20 minutes. Let the dip rest for 5 minutes before serving, but serve warm.

BLACK ORANGE SODA

A classic for the soda nerd – half Coca Cola and half Fanta orange. Actually really nice! (Cola Syrup, page 40, and Fizzy Orange Soda, page 82.)

BITTER SHANDY

In Britain's pleasant pub history you'll find many fine drinking traditions. One of them is shandy – a glass filled half with bitter or ale and the other half with fizzy lemonade.

There are plenty of variations on the drink – including alcohol-free versions – and many pubs make their own renditions, depending on what beer they have on tap and which kind of lemonade they stock. Others sell bottled shandy, which you can also buy in supermarkets. (Lemonade Syrup, page 25.)

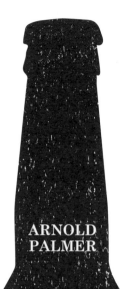

ARNOLD PALMER

If you like iced tea and lemonade, this is something you ought to try. Put half and half in a large glass filled with ice and you've got an Arnold Palmer. The name is said to derive from the American golfer with the same name, who apparently liked to gulp down the refreshing mix in the 1960s. (Iced Tea, page 68, and Classic Lemonade, page 53.)

CLARA DE LIMÓN AND CALIMUCHO

Spain's answer to shandy is Clara de limón. When you order in an ice-cold glass of this drink on a hot summer's evening you get a fresh mixture of light lager and sour lemon soda. The Spaniards have a habit of mixing both beer and wine with all sorts of things. Calimucho is another variety with red wine and cola, not a favourite of mine unfortunately, but Clara de limón is incredibly tasty! (Lemon Soda, page 78.)

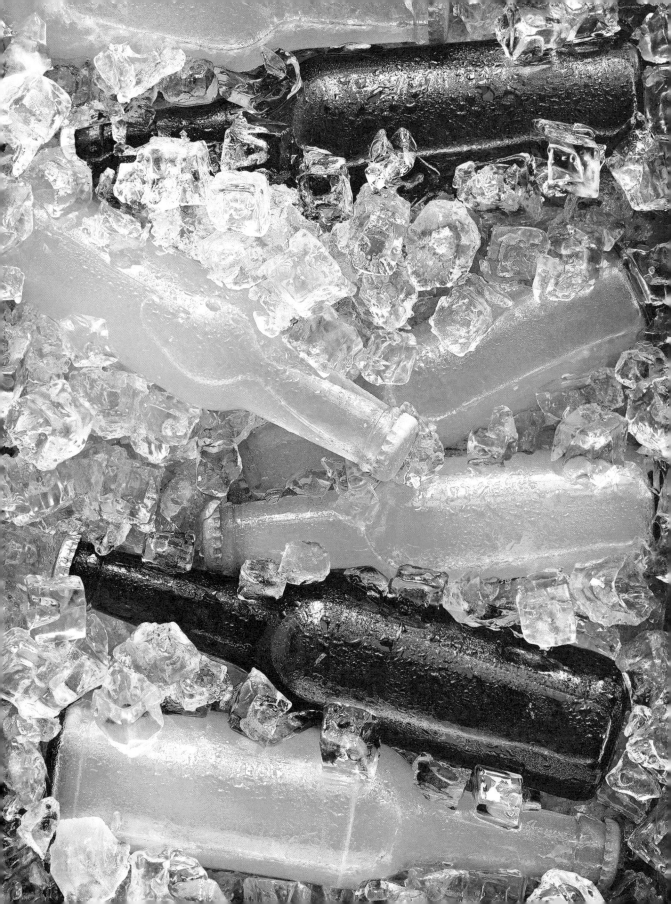

Fermented
DRINKS

I use two kinds of fermentation methods for soda. For one of them I ferment using yeast, which gives a finished result within 24 hours. The other method is a little more time consuming. For this, you leave the liquid to ferment naturally with help from bacteria culture made from ginger. A lacto-fermentation process is started and the soda is ready after about 1½ weeks. It will have small, nice and fizzy bubbles and a flavour and balance that is great to match with food or to use as a cocktail base.

The fermented tea drink kombucha is made using a third fermentation method. Here you use a kind of mushroom that's dropped into the liquid to be fermented, and which helps the lacto-fermentation process going and gives a lovely fizzy result.

The bubbles vary in all kinds of soda. When you use syrup and add sparkling water, the bubbles get quite large and climb up the walls of the glass. When you ferment using yeast, the bubbles get quite small but very 'lively', which sometimes give a nice prickly sensation in the mouth.

That the bubbles are different doesn't mean they contain different amounts of carbonic acid. Often, the naturally fermented soda is packed with carbonic acid, despite a less bubbly sensation in the mouth, and that's why these bottles should be opened very carefully.

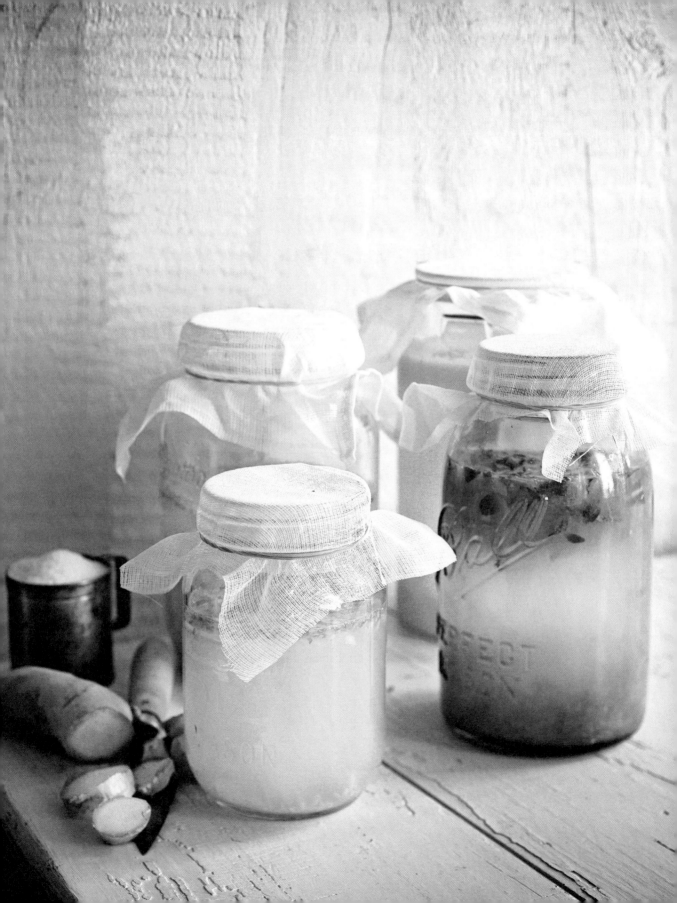

FERMENTING
with YEAST

To ferment soda using yeast is simple, but quantities are very important. The yeast is added to the liquid and will produce carbonic acid when the yeast bacteria eat the sugar. The longer the liquid ferments, the more carbonic acid there will be.

Only very small amounts of yeast are needed to make a good soda. If you add too much, the drink will just taste of yeast and, as too much yeast will produce too much carbonic acid, the bottles will explode under the pressure.

I use liquid champagne or cider yeast – Edelmans and Wyeast because they give the least amount of after-taste. After numerous tests using common baker's yeast and beer yeast I realised that there actually aren't any alternatives to the champagne yeast, since the soda simply wouldn't come out well in the end.

The best thing is always to brew soda in plastic PET bottles, so that you can monitor how much it has fermented. When the sides of the bottle become hard and taut, the soda has fermented and is full of carbonic acid. You can pour the soda into glass bottles after it's fermented and then place in the fridge to stall the fermentation process. So you don't lose all the fizz, you can place a chopstick in the funnel to make it bubble less when bottling the soda.

Swing-top bottles don't work very well as the soda will be under a lot of pressure when it's opened. When opening swing-top bottles it's difficult to do so carefully and there's a chance the cap will fly off. Bottles with screw caps or crown caps on the other hand, can be opened carefully, a little at a time, to avoid flying caps.

GRAPEFRUIT SODA

About 3 litres/5¼ pints/13¼ cups
1.5 litres/2½ pints/6½ cups water
225g/8oz/1½ cups granulated
  sugar
800ml/scant 1½ pints/3½ cups
  freshly squeezed grapefruit
  juice (about 6 grapefruits)
600ml/1 pint/generous 2½ cups
  freshly squeezed lemon juice
  (about 12 lemons)
a pinch of salt
scant ⅛ tsp liquid champagne or
  cider yeast

Bring 300ml/½ pint/1¼ cups of the water to the boil in a pan with the sugar. Leave to cool.

Squeeze the grapefruits and lemons, saving half of the pulp. Mix the juice with the pulp, syrup, salt and the rest of the water. Add the yeast and stir thoroughly. Pour into 2 PET bottles, leaving about 5cm/2in of air in the bottleneck. Squeeze the bottleneck to dent it, then put the cap on again. Leave to ferment at room temperature for 1–3 days.

When the dent in the bottle has straightened out and the plastic feels hard and taut, the soda is sufficiently carbonated. Pour into smaller bottles using a funnel and a chopstick (see left). Place in the fridge to stall the fermentation process.

LEMON SODA

Like a fizzy sour lemonade!

About 3 litres/5¼ pints/14¼ cups
300ml/½ pint/1¼ cups +
  1.5 litres/2½ pints/6½ cups
  water
200g/7oz/1 cup granulated sugar
600ml/1 pint/generous 2½ cups
  freshly squeezed lemon juice
  (about 12 lemons)
grated zest of 3 lemons
scant ⅛ tsp liquid champagne
  or cider yeast

Bring 300ml/½ pint/1¼ cups of water to the boil with the sugar in a pan. Mix with the lemon juice, zest and the rest of the water in a large bowl. Leave to cool.

Add the yeast and stir thoroughly so that the yeast is evenly spread throughout the liquid. Pour into 2 PET bottles, making sure there's about 5cm/2in of air in the bottleneck. Squeeze the bottleneck so it gets dented and put the cap on. Leave to ferment at room temperature for 1–3 days.

When the dent in the bottle has straightened out and the plastic feels hard and taut, the soda will be sufficiently carbonated. Pour into smaller bottles using a funnel and a chopstick (see left).

Place in the fridge to stall the fermentation process.

{
Storage
Keep the soda for a maximum of 4 weeks in the fridge. It will continue to slowly ferment, like a cold-risen dough when baking.
}

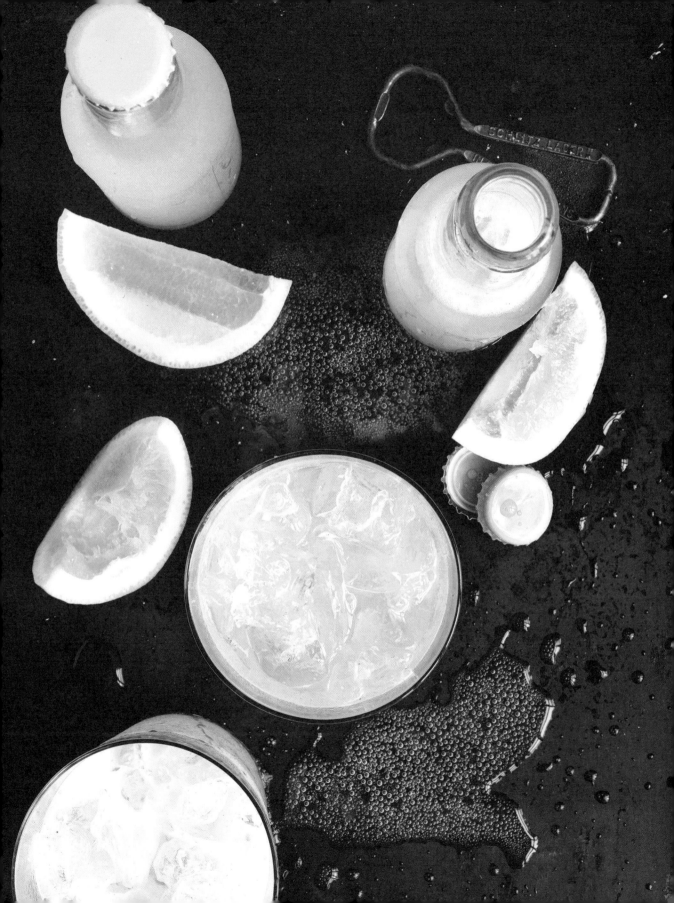

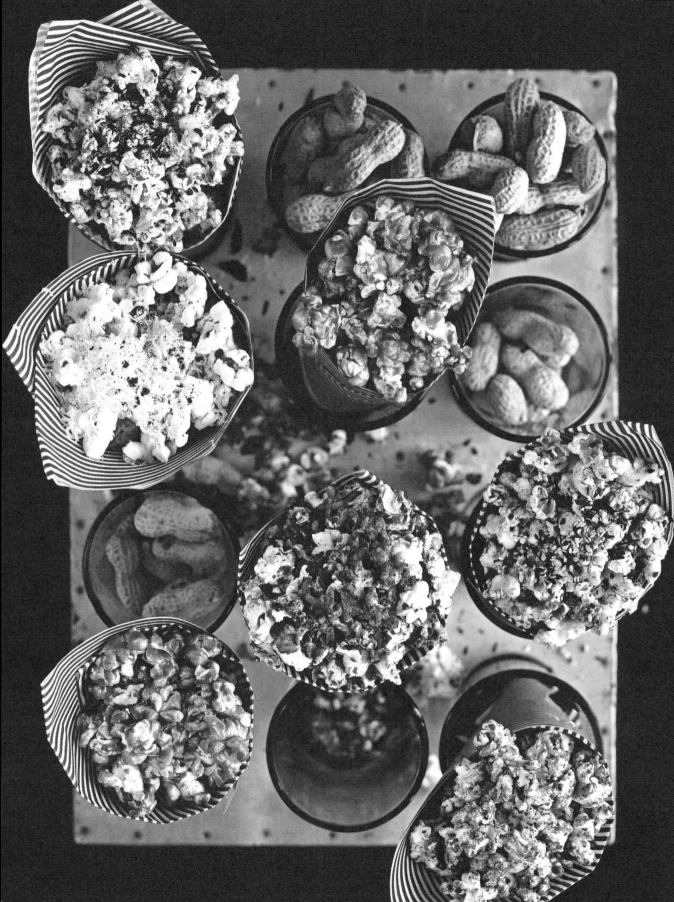

POPCORN

The perennial favourite – here are some extra-special flavours.

BASIC POPCORN

Popcorn without the microwave!

Serves 6–8
2 tbsp corn or rapeseed oil
200g/7oz/1 cup popping corn
½ tsp salt

Heat the oil in a large pan. Add the corn, put on the lid and shake gently to coat it in the oil. Leave over a low heat until the popcorn almost stops popping.

Remove the lid and add salt, then shake to spread it evenly.

SALTED CARAMEL POPCORN

Simply addictive – salty-caramel crispy popcorn.

Serves 6–8
225g/8oz/1½ cups granulated sugar
3 tbsp glucose syrup or liquid glucose
50g/1¾oz butter
3 tbsp whipping cream
1 tbsp bicarbonate of powder
½ tsp salt
1 batch Basic Popcorn (see above)

Preheat the oven to 100°C/50°F and line a baking tray with baking parchment. Melt the sugar and glucose syrup into a golden-brown caramel in a pan with a thick base. Add the butter and cream. Simmer until it has reached 125°C/257°F. Remove from the heat and quickly mix in the bicarbonate of soda and salt.

Place the popcorn in a large bowl (about 4 litres/7 pints/ 16 cups capacity), pour the caramel over the top and mix so that all the popcorn is covered. Pour out onto the prepared baking tray.

Dry in the middle of the oven for 1 hour, stirring every 15 minutes.

Leave to cool and store in an airtight bag or jar. The popcorn will keep for up to 3 weeks.

SESAME, NORI & WASABI POPCORN

This popcorn has a good kick from the wasabi and is packed with sesame seeds and algae: perfect to nibble with a refreshing soda.

Serves 6–8
1 nori leaf
1 egg white
2 tbsp wasabi paste
1 tsp sesame oil
1 tsp fish sauce
½ tbsp granulated sugar
1 tbsp clear honey
½ tsp salt
3–4 tbsp sesame seeds, preferable a mix of black and white
1 batch Basic Popcorn (see left)

Preheat the oven to 100°C/50°F and line a baking tray with baking parchment. Cut the nori leaf into small pieces. Mix the egg white, wasabi, sesame oil, fish sauce, sugar, honey, salt, sesame seeds and nori leaf in a large bowl (about 4 litres/ 7 pints/16 cups). Add the popcorn to the bowl and mix until it is all covered. Pour out the popcorn onto the prepared baking tray and dry

in the middle of the oven for about 1 hour, stirring every 15 minutes or so.

Leave to cool and season with more salt, if needed. Store in an airtight bag or jar. It will keep fresh for up to 3 weeks.

KIMCHI POPCORN

Popcorn with heat and a flavour explosion from kimchi. It will take a couple of hours in the oven, but it's worth it.

Serves 6–8
1 batch Basic Popcorn (see left)
2 tbsp kimchi paste
1 tbsp sriracha sauce (Thai chilli sauce)
1 tbsp sesame oil
½ tsp salt
120g/4¼oz kimchi

Preheat the oven to 100°C/50°F and line a baking tray with baking parchment. Drain the kimchi thoroughly using a sieve. Finely chop the kimchi and spread out onto the baking tray. Dry in the middle of the oven for about 30 minutes, stirring halfway through, then lower the heat to 70°C/150°F and cook for a further 1 hour, stirring every 15 minutes.

Mix the kimchi paste, sriracha, sesame oil and salt in a large bowl (about 4 litres/ 7 pints/16 cups) and stir the popcorn into the mixture, followed by the dried kimchi.

Dry in the middle of the oven for about 2 hours, stirring every 30 minutes. Leave to cool and season with more salt, if needed. It will keep fresh for up to 3 weeks.

SMOKY MAPLE POPCORN

The Spanish ground paprika, pimentón de la vera, can be added to many things for a nice smoky flavour. Here you also get heat from the paprika and chilli and a good amount of sweetness from the maple syrup.

Serves 6–8

2 tbsp maple syrup

1 egg white

1½ tsp Spanish smoked ground paprika (or other smoked ground paprika)

a small pinch of chilli flakes (heat of your choice)

1 tsp cumin

1 tsp onion powder

3 tbsp butter

a pinch of salt

1 batch Basic Popcorn (page 81)

Preheat the oven to 75°C/150°F and line a baking tray with baking parchment. Mix the maple syrup, egg white, spices, salt and melted butter in a large bowl (about 4 litres/ 7 pints/16 cups). Stir thoroughly so that the whole bowl gets sticky all round. Toss the popcorn around in the bowl until covered in the spices.

Pour the popcorn out onto the prepared baking tray. Dry in the middle of the oven for about 30 minutes, stirring after half the time.

Leave to cool and store in an airtight bag or jar. It will keep for up to 3 weeks.

PARMESAN & TRUFFLE POPCORN

Freshly popped, warm popcorn with tasty Parmesan and truffle oil. Try adding a couple of sprigs of fresh rosemary or sage when popping the corn – it makes a great combination.

Serves 6–8

1 batch Basic Popcorn (page 81)

1 pinch of white truffle oil

50g/1¾oz Parmesan cheese, finely grated

2 pinches of coarsely ground black pepper

Mix the freshly popped corn with the truffle oil, Parmesan and pepper. Serve immediately. This popcorn cannot be stored.

FIZZY ORANGE SODA

Forget about shop-bought brands – once you've tried this soda, you won't want to go back to factory-produced drinks. This soda tastes of pure orange with a nice acidity from the lemon.

About 3 litres/5¼ pints/14¼ cups

300ml/½ pint/1¼ cups + 150ml/ ¼ pint/scant ⅔ cup water

225g/8oz/1½ cups granulated sugar

200ml/7fl oz/scant 1 cup freshly squeezed lemon juice (about 3–4 lemons)

grated zest of 1 lemon

800ml/scant 1½ pints/3½ cups freshly squeezed orange juice (about 12 oranges)

grated zest of 4 oranges

scant ⅛ tsp liquid champagne or cider yeast

Bring 300ml/½ pint/1¼ cups water to the boil with the sugar in a pan. Mix with citrus juice, zest and the rest of the water in a large bowl. Leave to cool.

Add yeast and stir thoroughly so that the yeast is evenly spread throughout the liquid. Pour into two or three PET bottles, making sure there's about 5cm/2in of air in the bottleneck. Squeeze the bottleneck so that it is dented and put the cap on. Leave to ferment at room temperature for 1–2 days.

When the dent in the bottle has straightened out and the plastic feels hard and taut the soda is carbonated. Pour into smaller bottles using a funnel and a chopstick (see page 78).

Place in the fridge to stall the fermentation process.

Blood orange soda
When it's blood orange season from February to March, you can replace the normal oranges for sour blood-orange soda.

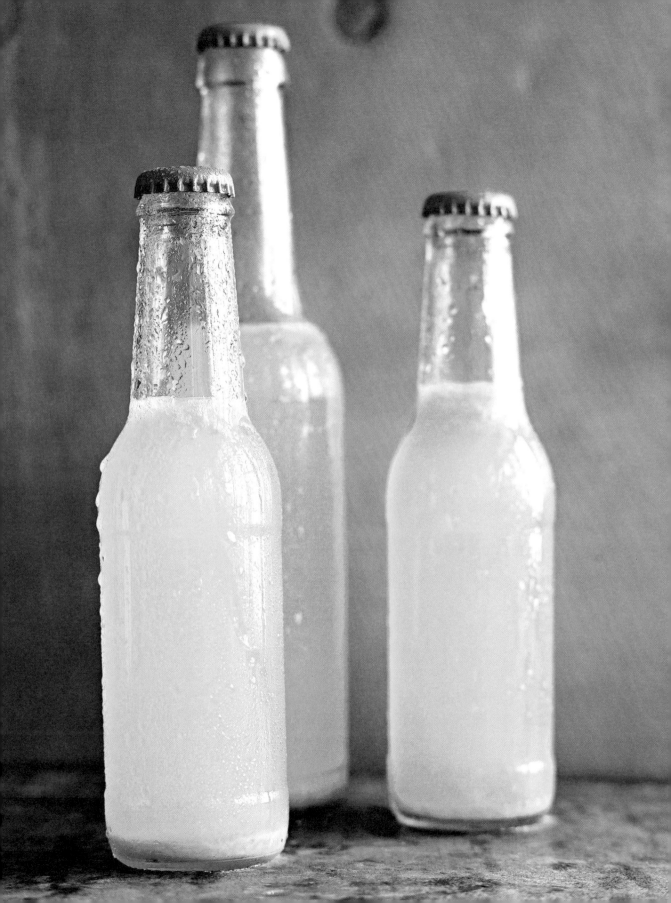

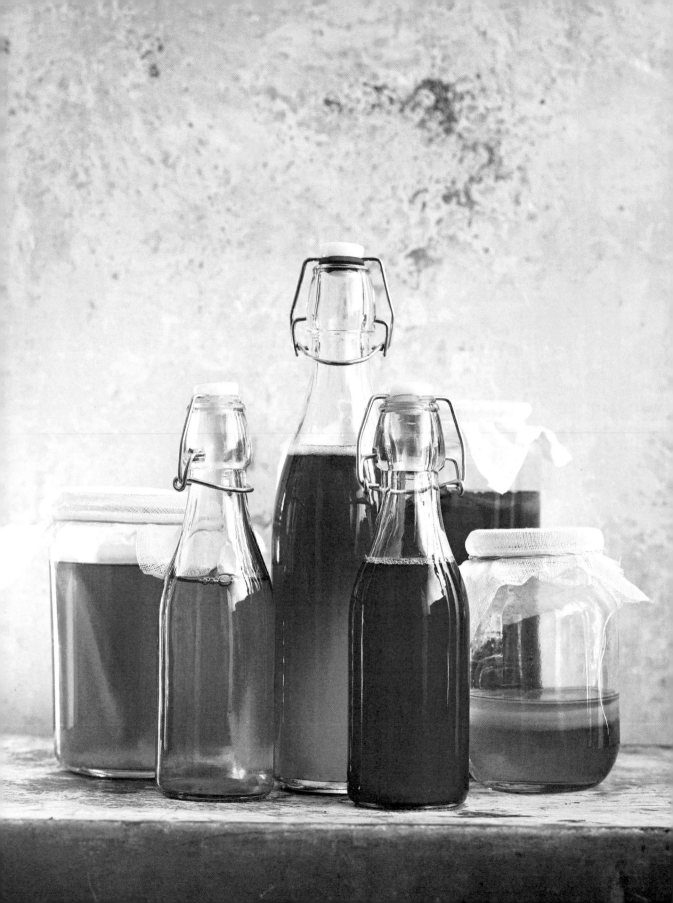

KOMBUCHA

The first time you taste homemade kombucha you'll be hooked. The fruity, flowery taste with vinegar acid is really tasty and properly refreshing.

Kombucha is tea that is fermented with the help of a flat, pancake-like mixture of yeasts called a mushroom, or SCOBY (symbiotic colony of bacteria and yeast). Kombucha has long been available as a health drink, but it has recently become more popular among the general public.

My 80-year-old relative from the north of Sweden, Anna-Stina, told me that when she was a little girl the grown-ups had a fine crystal bowl of kombucha in the middle of the living room. From time to time, the adults went and lifted up the mushroom, which was lying like a lid over the liquid, and slurped down a glass or two in the hope that the good bacteria culture would keep them healthy and strong. In the 1970s there was a kombucha mushroom hype associated with sourdough baking, commune living, green living and chilli con carne.

Now, the drink has gone from being a health drink to a trend drink that comes in lots of different flavours and variations and – without a doubt – it's here to stay.

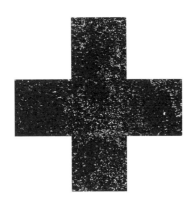

KOMBUCHA FIRST AID

1. APPEARANCE A scoby is transparent and jelly looking. It almost resembles a slimy jellyfish. The scoby grows thicker and thicker after every use and when it is very thick you can peel off a few layers to get a fresh mushroom again. The old layers you can use for growing a new scoby with the help of a small amount of fermented kombucha liquid.

2. THE POSITIONING OF THE SCOBY The scoby will either float on the surface of the liquid, or float sideways in the liquid – the fermentation will work either way. If the scoby floats sideways a scoby baby will be developed in the surface and you get an extra scoby to use or to give away to someone else.

3. SPOTS AND DEPOSITS It's normal that brown threads are developed on the underside of the scoby with deposits in the bottom of the liquid. The deposits can be strained off when bottling the finished drink, but you almost always have to count on some residue in the finished drink, also in the bottle.

If a hole appears in the scoby or if it develops dark brown spots this is completely normal and you can continue using it for fermenting. The brown spots and the threads you can carefully, and with clean hands, remove from the scoby when you start a new fermentation. If the scoby, on the other hand, turns black and perhaps gets some mould on it, it's time to get rid of it and grow a new one.

4. USE YOUR NOSE If the kombucha smells nice with a fresh vinegar smell there's nothing wrong with it. The further down the fermentation process, the more it will smell of vinegar. If the liquid gets too acidic you can start up a new batch and leave it to ferment for a slightly shorter time. However, it is important that the scoby is always stored in an acidic environment, since acid keeps the bad bacteria away. Always make sure that at least 10 percent of the liquid is made up of acidic kombucha from earlier batches. Taste the liquid after about a week to determine how acidic it should be. Some like it strongly acidic, almost like vinegar, and others prefer a bit sweeter and fruitier kombucha.

5. HOLIDAY AND REST If you're going on holiday and are worried about your scoby, you can let it rest. If you are away for less than 2 weeks you can store the scoby and brew a new batch of kombucha. If the liquid gets too acidic all you have to do is start on a fresh batch with the scoby and part of the liquid. If you are going away for longer you can take a chance and leave the scoby out in a very sweet tea (see Second batch, opposite). If it doesn't work you'll have to start again and grow a new scoby from a bottle of kombucha you might have saved in the fridge from an earlier batch. Just like with sourdough, it's possible to leave the scoby to rest for a little longer in the fridge in a few tablespoons of kombucha. It might take a little longer to get the fermentation started after the rest.

6. STORING Store fermenting kombucha at room temperature (20–25°C/60–77°F). When it has been bottled and finished fermenting it's stored in the fridge to stall the fermentation process. If it keeps fermenting for longer at room temperature, there's a chance the bottles will explode from the pressure.

7. BOTTLES Use small PET bottles or glass bottles with swing tops so they are easy to open and check when the drink is fizzy enough. If you use PET bottles the drink is ready when the plastic is taut and hard. With glass bottles you'll simply have to open a bottle after about 2 days to check how fizzy the drink has managed to get. I prefer to bottle up into several small bottles (about 240ml/8fl oz/1 cup) to avoid having to have opened bottles in the fridge that lose some of their fizz once opened.

HOW DO I GET HOLD OF A SCOBY?

To get started with kombucha fermentation you'll need a scoby. The easiest way to get hold of one is to ask someone who ferments kombucha if they've got a scoby going spare, just like when you get a bit of sourdough starter from someone. Otherwise the alternative is to get one from a home-brew store or online.

You can also grow your own scoby with the help from un-pasteurised bought kombucha, or finished kombucha that you've been given by someone. Then you simply pour the ready-made drink into a clean glass jar and cover with muslin fastened with a rubber band. Then you leave it for 2–4 weeks and wait for a scoby to be developed on the surface. The scoby, together with some of the liquid, can then be used for making your own kombucha.

KOMBUCHA

You can make kombucha from both black and green tea. I often make mine from ordinary Earl Grey, as I like the fact there's a taste of the tea in the finished drink. If you use green tea the taste will be mild and neutral, which is very good when making flavoured kombucha.

If you start from scratch with a scoby and the liquid it comes with it's best to start from the beginning with the first batch below.

Later when you've bottled your first batch of finished kombucha (see point 7 in the second batch) and want to continue with yet another batch you can get started on the second batch straightaway and in this way always have kombucha fermenting away in the kitchen.

BASIC KOMBUCHA

FIRST BATCH
500ml/17fl oz/generous 2 cups water
1 tsp black or green tea leaves
50g/1¾oz/¼ cup granulated sugar
200ml/7fl oz/scant 1 cup finished kombucha or kombucha starter (the liquid that you get when buying a scoby)
1 scoby

1. Bring half the water and the tea to the boil in a large pan.
2. Remove from the heat and stir in the sugar. Leave to steep for 30 minutes, covered with a lid or covered with a thin tea towel or muslin.
3. Run the liquid through a fine

sieve into a glass jar that holds 1 litre/1¾ pints/4⅓ cups.
4. Add the rest of the cold water and leave to cool, covered.
5. Check that the liquid has cooled to room temperature, then add the kombucha or kombucha starter.
6. With clean hands, add the scoby, preferably on the surface with the completely smooth and shiny side facing upwards. If the scoby is very thin and newly produced you can just add it to the liquid and then carefully spread it out so that it doesn't form into a lump.
7. Leave to stand, covered with a thin tea towel or muslin fastened with a rubber band, at room temperature for 1–2 weeks. You can sometimes see there are small bubbles in the kombucha when it has fermented for some time, then you'll know for sure that the fermentation process is working as it should.
8. After 1–2 weeks it's time to mix the first batch with the second batch to get an even bigger batch.

SECOND BATCH
3 litres/5¼ pints/13¼ cups water
2 tbsp black or green tea leaves
200g/7oz/generous 1 cup granulated sugar
300ml/½ pint/1¼ cups kombucha (from batch 1)
1 scoby

1. Bring half the water to the boil in a large pan together with the tea.
2. Remove from the heat and

stir in the sugar. Leave to steep for 30 minutes, covered with a lid, and then drain the tea leaves off through a fine sieve. Strain the liquid into a glass jar that holds 4 litres/ 7 pints/16 cups.
3. Add the remaining water.
4. Leave to cool, covered with a thin tea towel or muslin. It's important that the liquid is cooled down completely, if it's not the scoby will die in the hot liquid.
5. When the liquid is at room temperature, add the kombucha from the first batch and carefully place the scoby on top of the liquid.
6. Cover with a tea towel fastened with a rubber band. Leave to stand for 1–2 weeks at room temperature. Taste the liquid after 1 week and decide how acidic you want it – the longer it stands, the more acidic it will get.
7. When the liquid has fermented for 1–2 weeks it's ready to be bottled. Prepare a new second batch that gets time to cool down before bottling so that the scoby can be transferred over once the finished liquid is filled into the bottles. Make sure you save 300ml/½ pint/1¼ cups liquid for the new batch together with the scoby.
8. Use small PET bottles or glass bottles with swing caps. Make sure the bottles are sterilised and then strain in the kombucha using a sieve and a funnel. Fill until you're left with about 5cm/2in air in the bottlenecks. Put the caps on the bottles.
9. Leave to stand at room temperature for 1–5 days to get the drink properly carbonated. If you are using PET bottles, feel the bottle neck – if the plastic is taut and hard it's time to put them in the fridge. If you are using glass bottles you'll have to open a bottle after a couple of days to check how carbonated it is. Sometimes small deposits will appear at the top of the bottle, but that doesn't matter. You'll just have to strain the kombucha before drinking it.

FLAVOURED KOMBUCHA

Kombucha brewed with fruit and berries is like a sour carbonated lemonade with vinegar acid instead of citrus. Raspberries and peach are favourites, but it's fun to try different kinds of fruit and berries in the hunt for the prefect kombucha. Try leaving herbs like thyme, sage or rosemary to ferment together with the liquid to give it a deeper flavour.

1. Make the kombucha as usual to step 7 in the second batch (when it's time to bottle).
2. Prepare a new second batch and allow it to cool down. Save the scoby and 300ml/ ½ pint/1¼ cups of the liquid for the new batch.
3. Mix the fermented kombucha (without scoby) with 200g/7oz room-temperature, mashed or puréed fruit or berries in a large glass jar.
4. Cover with muslin fastened with a rubber band and leave to stand for 1–2 days.
5. Strain and bottle, leaving about 5cm/2in of air in the bottleneck.
6. Leave the bottles to stand at room temperature for 1–3 days to carbonate.
7. Place in the fridge to stall the fermentation process. It will stay fresh in the fridge for up to a month.

TASTY FLAVOURINGS

Of course you can vary the tea varieties in kombucha – classic Earl Grey, neutral green tea, flowery black tea, jasmine or vanilla and citrus. Berries, fruits and herbs you can mix and match just as you please until you find a favourite. The ultimate flavour for me is lingonberry and lemon zest. Remember that flavoured kombucha will often carbonate a bit more quickly than neutral kombucha.

Blueberries
Cranberries
Ginger
Lemon balm
Lemon or lime zest
Lemongrass
Mint
Passionfruit and lemon zest
Pineapple and lime zest
Orange flower water
Orange zest
Raspberries or strawberries
Rosewater
Sea buckthorn

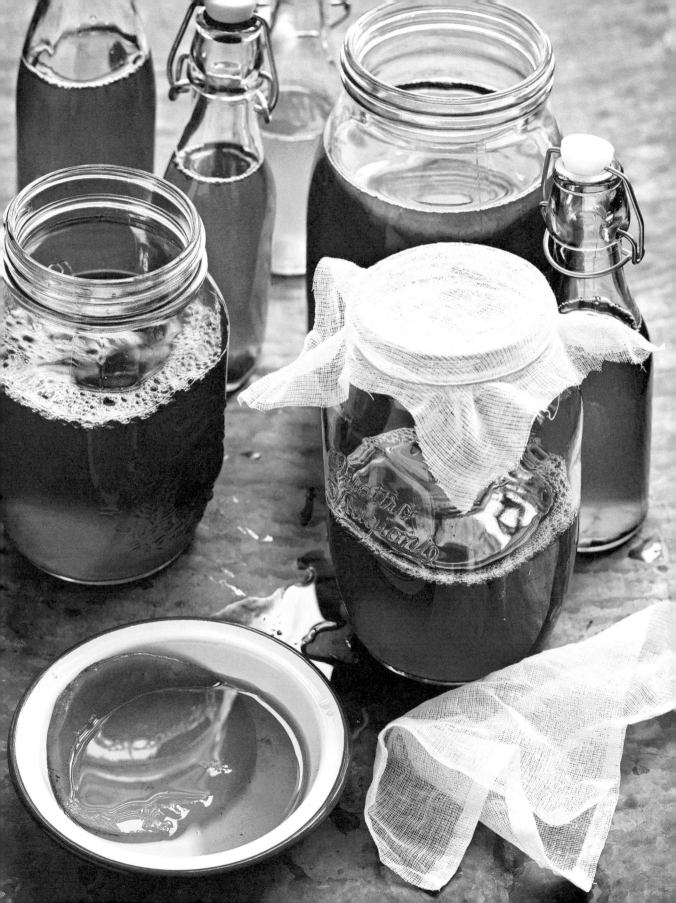

NATURALLY *fermented* SODA

Developing soda with natural fermentation can be regarded as the soda nerd's answer to sourdough baking. Lacto-fermentation doesn't only work for pickles or sauerkraut but also for soda. To get carbonic acid in a drink completely naturally without yeast or a soda maker, you mix together a soda culture. The soda culture is made of three ingredients: water, sugar and some kind of root (for example dandelion root or ginger). I use ginger as it gives a nice flavour to the finished drink and you can also get hold of it everywhere all year around.

In the US, soda culture made from ginger is called a ginger bug, but I call it soda starter or soda culture. This kind of natural fermentation is easy to use, but demands gentle handling, just like sourdough. You care tenderly for the culture for a few days and then mix it with a fruit or berry juice of your choice in a large glass jar. The liquid is left to ferment, covered with muslin, for yet another few days and then it's time to bottle it. The culture should be fed regularly and if you are going away you have to leave it in the fridge to rest and then get it started again when you come home. The drink is partly carbonated during the fermentation process, but it's when the liquid is bottled that the carbonic acid is trapped in the bottle and gives the drink a properly fizzy character. It might sound a little tricky, but just like with sourdough it's very straightforward once you've got started!

A successful natural soda fermentation gives an incredibly tasty result with a real depth and a sour freshness. You can never guarantee that you will get the same flavour in the soda each time, since a lot of different factors have an effect on the fermentation process – how ripe the fruit is, the room temperature – simply the circumstances the liquid is in at that moment. But that's a part of the charm with homemade beverages. The soda varies in taste in the same way that wine varies in character depending on climate and weather conditions.

If you're unlucky enough to over-ferment the soda, it won't taste very nice. It will smell and taste of stale yeast, which is not what you are after! When you ferment using whole berries or with a lot of fruit pulp in the liquid, the fermentation process will normally speed up, since there's quite a lot of sugar both from the fruit and from any added sugar that the yeast bacteria like to eat. Stir several times a day to mix the fruit and to get the bacteria to work. When you see bubbles in the liquid and hear a fizzing sound it's important to bottle the drink immediately, don't wait – or you'll only regret it.

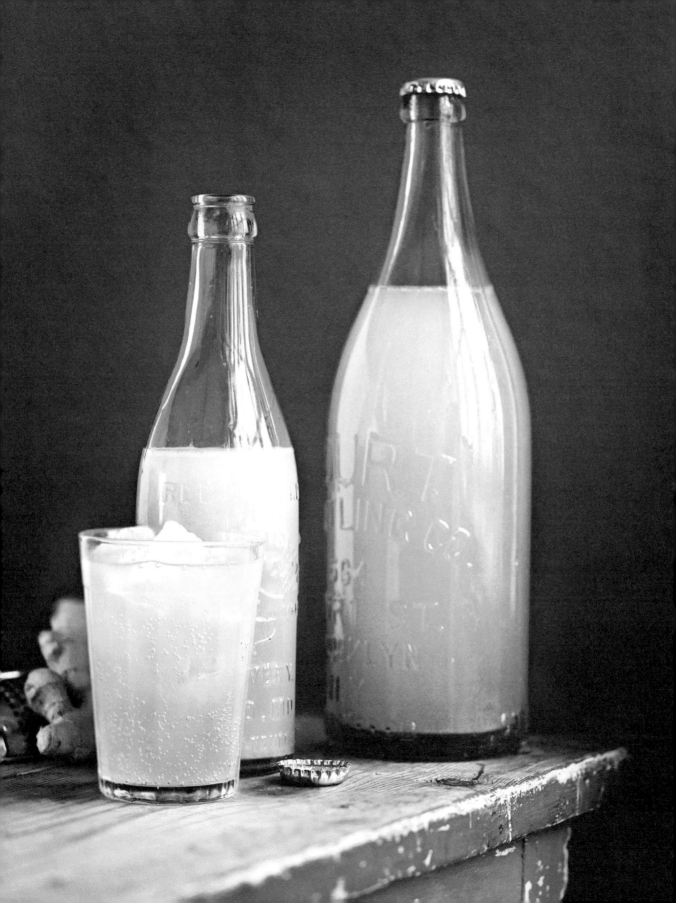

SODA CULTURE
– GINGER STARTER
'GINGER BUG'

It's relatively quick to get a soda culture started. In contrast to the kombucha mushroom, which you don't want to lose as it's a bit tricky to get hold of a new one, you only have to mix together some water, sugar and ginger to get a new soda starter. I almost always brew soda made from freshly made soda culture, as I find it a bit difficult to keep more than one jar among all the spices, cookery books and tools in my kitchen. Besides, I think the finished soda feels a bit fresher both in smell and flavour if it's made from fresh soda culture.

500ml/17fl oz/generous 2 cups water
2 tbsp finely grated ginger
1 tbsp granulated sugar
1 tbsp Demerara sugar

1. Mix all the ingredients together in a sterilised glass jar.
2. Cover with thin fabric fastened with a rubber band so that the liquid can breathe in the jar.
3. Leave the jar to stand for 1–4 days. I find 2 days tends to be enough, but it all depends on how the culture is thriving in your kitchen. I keep the jar on top of the fridge where it's a bit warmer and then the culture usually gets started straight away.
4. Stir the liquid 1–3 times every day and add 1 tsp of finely grated ginger, ½ tsp granulated sugar and ½ tsp Demerara sugar once a day.
5. When you see bubbles on the surface of the liquid and hear a fizzing sound when you stir it, the ginger starter is ready. The liquid is normally a bit cloudy, but if it smells clean everything is in order. Now it's ready to be used!
6. To keep the starter active, it will need to be fed regularly, just like a sourdough. Feed it as before with 1 tsp sugar and 1 tsp finely grated ginger each day.
7. You can also leave the starter to 'rest' in the fridge. Place a lid on the jar and leave the culture in the fridge. Feed it with 1 tsp finely grated ginger, ½ tsp granulated sugar and ½ tsp Demerara sugar once a week. To wake it up again, take it out of the fridge. When it's reached room temperature it can be fed once a day.

General rule when naturally fermenting soda
(exceptions can occur):
About 3 tbsp soda culture to 1 litre/1¾ pints/4⅓ cups liquid.

Stir
Stir the fermenting soda 2–3 times a day. The soda culture 'likes' to be stirred, it gets the fermentation process going a bit quicker and reduces the risk for a failed fermentation and mould.

Ready?
If you use plastic bottles you can squeeze the bottle at the top before putting on the cap. Now it's easy to see when the drink has finished carbonating. If the plastic is hard and taut, the soda is ready.

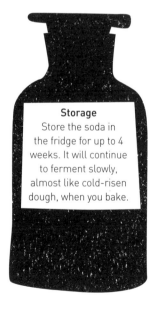

Storage
Store the soda in the fridge for up to 4 weeks. It will continue to ferment slowly, almost like cold-risen dough, when you bake.

GINGER BEER

One of my favourites in the book, there's nothing as nice as a perfectly balanced ginger beer with a good amount of acidity, freshness and a sting of ginger.

About 3 litres/5¼ pints/13¼ cups
3 litres/5¼ pints/13¼ cups water
200g/7oz/1 cup granulated sugar
150g/5½oz/¾ cup Demerara sugar
200g/7oz chopped fresh root ginger
200ml/7fl oz/scant 1 cup freshly
    squeezed lemon juice (about
    3–4 lemons)
100ml/3½fl oz/scant ½ cup Soda
    Culture (see opposite)

Bring 600ml/1 pint/generous 2½ cups water to the boil with the sugar and ginger. Leave to simmer for about 5 minutes. Mix with the remaining water in a glass jar that holds 4 litres/7 pints/16 cups and leave to cool.

Mix with the lemon juice, then add the soda culture through a sieve. Cover with muslin fastened with a rubber band. Leave to stand at room temperature for 4–7 days, stirring 2–3 times a day.

Check the taste after 4 days. The longer it stands, the drier it will get, but don't let the soda over-ferment – it should still smell of fresh ginger.

Strain and bottle in sterilised PET or glass bottles (300ml/ ½ pint/1¼ cup), leaving about 5cm/2in of air in each bottle. Put on the caps and leave at room temperature for about 1–2 days to carbonate. Transfer to the fridge so that the fermentation process is stalled.

RED CURRANT & CHERRY SODA

This gives you a dry soda that makes a decent alternative to red wine. The sour currants and cherries are almost like a lighter North Italian table wine.

About 3 litres/5¼ pints/13¼ cups
2.5 litres/4¼ pints/10 cups water
200g/7oz/1 cup granulated sugar
200g/7oz red or black currants
200g/7oz cherries
pared zest of 1 lemon
200ml/7fl oz/scant 1 cup freshly
    squeezed lemon juice (about
    3–4 lemons)
150ml/¼ pint/scant ⅔ cup Soda
    Culture (see opposite)

Boil 1 litre/1¾ pints/4⅓ cups of the water with the sugar and berries. Pour into a large glass jar that holds 4 litres/ 7 pints/16 cups and add the remaining cold water, the lemon zest and juice. Cover with muslin and leave to cool to room temperature.

Add the soda culture through a sieve and stir thoroughly. Cover with muslin fastened with a rubber band. Leave to stand at room temperature for 4–7 days. Stir 2–3 times a day.

Check the taste after 4 days to see how sweet the soda is. The longer it stands, the drier it will get since the sugar is 'eaten up' by the culture. But don't let the soda over-ferment – it should still smell fresh.

Strain the liquid and bottle into sterilised PET or glass bottles. Don't fill all the way up but leave about 5cm/2in of air in each bottle. Put on the caps

and leave at room temperature for 1–2 days so that the drink gets carbonated. Transfer to the fridge so that the fermentation process is stalled.

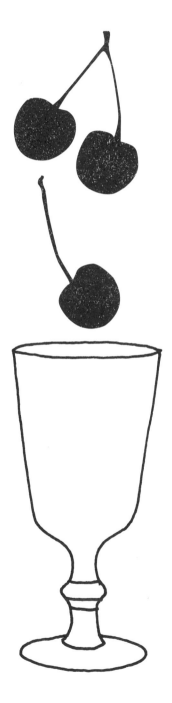

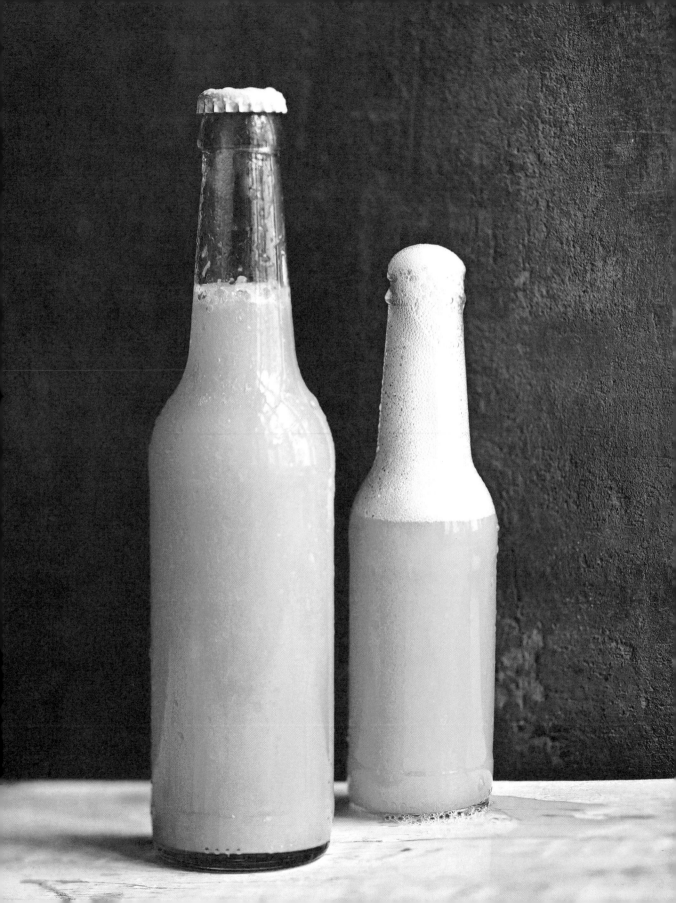

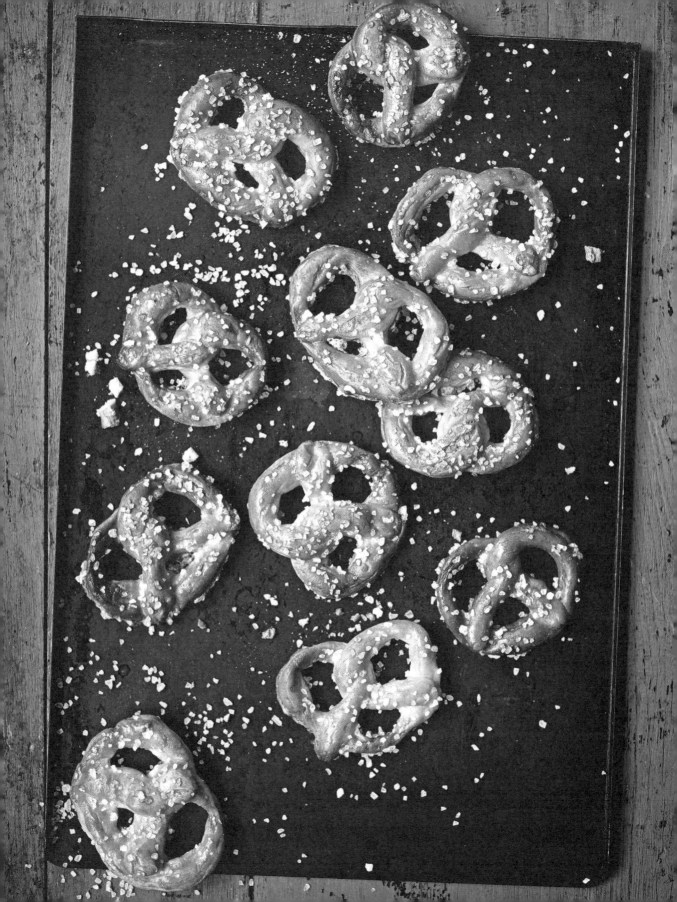

'CAMPARI' – GRAPEFRUIT & HERB SODA

My favourite among the fermented beverages in this book, the end result is like a nice Campari drink with bitterness and herbiness. Try mixing the soda with a shot of gin – oh, yes!

About 3.5 litres/6 pints/14 cups
800ml/scant 1½ pints/3½ cups
 freshly squeezed grapefruit
 juice (about 8 grapefruits)
grated zest of 1 grapefruit
500ml/17fl oz/generous
 2 cups freshly squeezed
 pink grapefruit juice
 (about 5 grapefruits)
250ml/9fl oz/generous 1 cup
 freshly squeezed lemon juice
 (about 5–6 lemons)
2.5 litres/4¼ pints/10 cups water
200g/7oz/1 cup granulated sugar
25g/1oz thyme sprigs
6 sage leaves
100ml/3½fl oz/scant ½ cup Soda
 Culture (see page 92)

Squeeze the citrus fruits. Save 100g/3¾oz of the pulp in the liquid. Peel 1 grapefruit with a knife or peeler so that you get a lot of the white peel included too, as this will give extra bitterness to the drink.

Boil 1 litre/1¾ pints/4⅓ cups of the water together with the sugar. Pour into a large glass jar that holds 4 litres/7 pints/16 cups and add the remaining cold water. Add the citrus juices, zest, pulp and herbs. Cover with muslin and leave to cool to room temperature.

Add the soda culture through a sieve and stir thoroughly.

Cover with muslin fastened with a rubber band. Leave to stand at room temperature for 3–5 days. Stir 2–3 times a day.

The pulp will float on the surface of the liquid and get more and more bubbly the longer the fermentation process continues. The pulp contains a lot of sugar that the yeast bacteria like so this soda usually ferments relatively quickly.

Check the taste after 3 days to see how sweet the soda is. The longer it stands, the drier it will get since the sugar is 'eaten up' by the culture. But don't let the soda over-ferment – it should still smell fresh. If you hear a clear fizzing sound when you stir, it is time to bottle the soda. Strain the liquid and bottle into sterilised PET or glass bottles. Don't fill all the way up but leave about 5cm/2in of air in each bottle. Leave the soda at room temperature for 1–2 days so that it is fully carbonated. Transfer to the fridge so that the fermentation process is stalled. (See photograph on page 94.)

LINGONBERRY & ORANGE BLOSSOM SODA

If you can't get lingonberries, use cranberries instead.

About 3 litres/5¼ pints/13¼ cups
2.5 litres/4¼ pints/10 cups water
225g/8oz/1¼ cups granulated sugar
450g/1lb lingonberries or
 cranberries
1 tsp orange blossom water
250ml/9fl oz/generous 1 cup
 freshly squeezed lemon juice
 (about 5–6 lemons)
100ml/3½fl oz/scant ½ cup soda
 culture

Boil 1 litre/1¾ pints/4⅓ cups of the water with the sugar and berries. Pour into a glass jar that holds 4 litres/7 pints/16 cups and add the remaining water. Add the orange blossom water and lemon juice. Cover with muslin and leave to cool to room temperature.

Add the soda culture through a sieve and stir thoroughly. Cover with muslin fastened with a rubber band. Leave to stand at room temperature for 4–7 days. Stir 2–3 times a day.

Check the taste after 4 days. The longer it stands, the drier it will get, but don't let it over-ferment – it should still smell fresh. If you hear a fizzing sound when you stir, it is ready to bottle. Strain and bottle into sterilised PET or small glass bottles, leaving about 5cm/2in of air in each bottle. Leave at room temperature for 1–2 days so that it carbonates. Transfer to the fridge so that the fermentation process is stalled.

PRETZELS

Pretzel or bretzel? In the US this salty snack is called pretzel and in Germany where it is said to have originated from it's called bretzel. To get the characteristic dark and shiny surface, the dough knots are dipped in simmering water mixed with baking powder and sugar.

It's possible to make pretzels in all kinds of sizes, everything from mini-mini to the larger size of the soft pretzels that you buy on the streets in New York. The latter version is served with a good dollop of American bright yellow mustard that you can dip the pretzel in while you're strolling down the street.

This recipe is suited for large or small snack-sized pretzels, which are enjoyed on their own. It's a bit more fiddly to do the small ones, but they're easier to get crispy than the larger ones. If you want to make them even smaller, just go for it, but as mentioned, it gets quite fiddly!

Makes 40 or 80

12.5g/½ oz fresh yeast
250g/9oz/generous 1 cup water
1 tbsp light muscovado sugar
½ tsp salt
250g/9oz/2 cups plain flour
1 tbsp rapeseed oil
1.5 litres/2½ pints/6½ cups boiling water
2 tbsp bicarbonate of soda
2 tbsp light muscovado sugar
1 egg, beaten
1–2 tbsp medium coarse sea salt or salt flakes

Crumble the yeast into a bowl and mix with water, sugar and salt. Stir until the yeast has dissolved in the liquid. Add the flour and work into a smooth dough. Knead for about 5 minutes on a worktop. The dough should be thoroughly springy and smooth.

Grease a bowl with a little oil and place the dough in the bowl. Flip it over so that the dough gets covered in oil. Cover the bowl with clingfilm and leave to rise for about 1 hour.

Split the dough into 2 halves and roll into long sausages. Cut each length into 20 or 40 pieces, depending on which size you are making. Grease an oven tray with a little more oil.

Roll the dough pieces into thin strips, about 30–35cm/ 12–14in long (shorter for small pretzels and longer for large ones), and form every strip into a knot. Make sure you press down the dough ends properly so that they don't fall off the pretzel. Place the pretzels on the oiled tray and leave to rise for 30 minutes, covered with clingfilm. (Clingfilm will keep the moisture in and is used instead of a tea towel.) Preheat the oven to 170°C/350°F and line a baking sheet with baking parchment.

Bring the water to the boil in a pan, then pour it into a flameproof stainless oven dish. Add the baking powder and sugar to the water. Leave the water to simmer in the dish on top of the stove. Add the pretzels in batches and simmer for about 2–3 minutes, depending on size, keeping them immersed in the water.

Take out the pretzels with a slotted spoon and place them on the prepared baking sheets. Leave them to dry up a little.

Brush the pretzels with beaten egg and sprinkle with salt. Bake in the middle of the oven for about 30-40 minutes.

Leave to cool on a wire rack. Store in an airtight jar or bag. If you like your pretzels a little softer you can take them out after about 20–30 minutes. (See photograph on page 95.)

ELDERFLOWER CHAMPAGNE

Naturally fermented elderflower champagne without a ginger soda culture, here the fermentation gets started by the elderflower heads and sugar.

About 2 litres/3½ pints/8 cups
20 elderflower heads
150ml/¼ pint/scant ⅔ cup freshly squeezed lemon juice (about 2–3 lemons)
finely grated zest of 2–3 lemons
200g/7oz/1 cup granulated sugar
1½ tbsp cider vinegar
2 litres/3½ cups/10 cups water

Clean the elderflower heads. Peel the lemons with a paring knife or a vegetable peeler and make sure to only get the yellow part of the zest and no white, which will give a bitter taste to the drink. Squeeze the juice to give 150ml/¼ pint/⅔ cup.

Mix together the lemon zest and juice with sugar, vinegar and water in a large bowl. Add the elderflowers. Cover with muslin secured with rubber bands. Leave to stand at room temperature for 1–2 days.

Strain through a straining cloth or muslin and bottle into plastic or glass bottles. Leave about 5cm/2in of air in the bottlenecks. Leave the bottles to stand at room temperature for 3–5 days.

Check one of the bottles after 2 days to see if it has become carbonated. Place in the fridge once carbonated to stall the fermentation process.

BLUEBERRY & LAVENDER FIZZ

About 3.5 litres/6 pints/14 cups
2.5 litres/ cold water
500g/1lb 2oz blueberries
200g/7oz dried lavender
200g/7oz/1 cup cane sugar
450ml/¾ pint/scant 2 cups freshly squeezed lime juice (about 12 limes)
150ml/¼ pint/ scant ⅔ cup Soda Culture (see page 92)

Bring 1 litre/1¾ pints/4⅓ cups of the water to the boil together with the blueberries, lavender and sugar in a pan.

Put the lime juice in a glass jar that holds at least 4 litres/7 pints/16 cups. Remove the blueberry liquid from the heat and add another 1.5 litres/2½ pints/6½ cups of cold water. Pour into the glass jar. Cover with muslin and leave to cool to room temperature.

Stir in the soda culture and cover with muslin. Leave to stand at room temperature for 3–5 days. Stir 2–3 times a day.

Check the taste after 3 days to see how sweet the soda is. The longer it stands, the drier it will get since the sugar is 'eaten up' by the culture. But don't let the soda over-ferment – it should still smell fresh. If you hear a fizzing sound when you stir it, it's ready to bottle.

Strain the liquid and bottle into sterilised PET or small glass bottles. Don't fill all the way up but leave about 5cm/2in of air in each bottle.

Leave the soda at room temperature for 1–2 days until carbonated. Transfer to the fridge to halt fermentation.

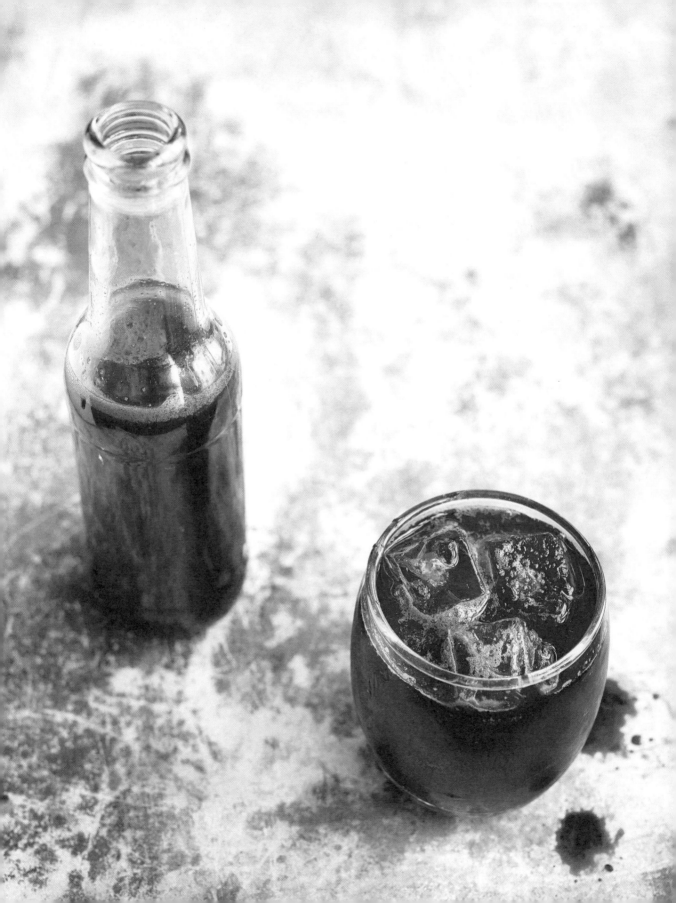

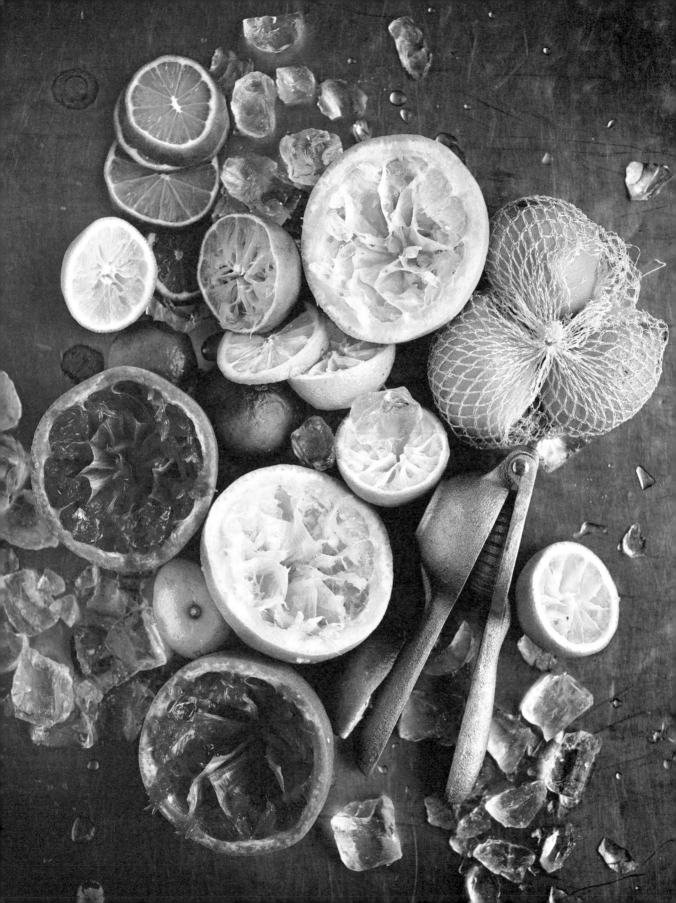

TROPICAL ORANGE & PASSION CRUSH

About 3 litres/5¼ pints/13¼ cups
800ml/scant 1½ pints/3½ cups
    freshly squeezed orange juice
    (about 12 oranges)
finely grated zest of 3 oranges
150ml/¼ pint/scant ⅔ cup passion
    fruit juice (frozen or freshly
    squeezed)
150ml/¼ pint/scant ⅔ cup freshly
    squeezed lime juice (about
    4–5 limes)
2 litres/3½ pints/8 cups water
200g/7oz/1 cup granulated sugar
100ml/3½fl oz/scant ½ cup Soda
    Culture (see page 92)

Squeeze the citrus fruits and strain off the pulp. Spoon the flesh from the passion fruits and run the juice through a sieve.

Boil 1 litre/1¾ pints/4⅓ cups of the water with the sugar. Pour into a large glass jar that holds 4 litres/7 pints/16 cups and add 1 litre/1¾ pints/4⅓ cups of cold water. Add the passion fruit juice and citrus juice. Cover with muslin and leave to cool to room temperature.

Add the soda culture through a sieve and stir thoroughly. Cover with muslin fastened with a rubber band. Leave to stand at room temperature for 3–5 days. Stir 2–3 times a day.

The pulp will float on the surface of the liquid and get increasingly bubbly. The pulp contains a lot of sugar that the yeast bacteria like so this soda usually ferments relatively quickly.

Check the taste after 3 days to see how sweet the soda is.

The longer it stands, the drier it will get since the sugar is 'eaten up' by the culture. But don't let the soda over-ferment, it should still smell fresh. If you hear a clear fizzing sound when you stir, it is ready to bottle. Strain and bottle into sterilised PET or glass bottles, leaving about 5cm/2in of air in each bottle. Leave at room temperature for 1–2 days so that it gets carbonated. Transfer to the fridge to stall fermentation.

ROASTED ALMONDS

Nice to crunch with a glass of cold Clara de limón (half lemon Fanta and half light lager, see page 74). In Spain they use the salt-roasted Marcona almonds from Catalonia. They are flatter and rounder than the almonds we're used to and the flavour has a good hint of bitter almond – the Rolls Royce of almonds in other words. If you just want to get going without any fancy details, normal almonds will also be nice for this recipe.

4 snack portions
200ml/7fl oz/¾ cup water
2 tbsp salt
200g/7oz/1½ cups almonds,
    preferably Marcona almonds

Preheat the oven to 200°C/400°F. Bring the water and salt to the boil in a pan. Add the almonds to the pan and leave to stand for about 10 minutes. Strain off the water and spread the almonds out on a baking tray. Roast in the middle of the oven for about 15 minutes. Stir after half the time. Serve.

Smoky almonds
If you want a smoky flavour on your almonds you can mix them with 1 tsp smoked ground paprika before they go into the oven. For a Tex-Mex flavour you can use ½ tsp ground paprika and ½ tsp cumin instead.

ROOT BEER

Flavouring soda with roots, leaves, bark, spices and herbs goes back a long way, and one example is American root beer, which gets its typical brown colour from unrefined sugar. The distinctive flavour varies depending on the recipe and – just like with spaghetti Bolognese – everyone thinks their own family recipe is the best. The basic rule is to brew from the root sarsaparilla and sassafras to get the unique flavour.

If you are used to shop-bought root beer, you might get a shock from the flavour of my version as they don't resemble each other much at all. But look at this as something new and very tasty!

About 3 litres/5¼ pints/13¼ cups
3 litres/5¼ pints/13¼ cups water
3 tbsp raisins
3 tbsp finely chopped ginger
100g/3½oz sarsaparilla root
3 tbsp sassafras root
2 tbsp hops
½ tbsp dandelion root
1 tbsp juniper berries, coarsely crushed
1 cinnamon stick (about 4cm/1½in)
300g/10½oz/1¾ cups dark muscovado sugar
1 tsp citric acid
150ml/¼ pint/scant ⅔ cup Soda Culture (see page 92)

Mix half the water with the raisins, ginger and all the spices. Bring to the boil and simmer for about 5 minutes. Mix with the sugar and citric acid. Pour into a large glass jar that holds 4 litres/ 7 pints/16 cups and add the remaining water. Cover with muslin fastened with a rubber band and leave to cool.

Add the soda culture through a sieve and stir thoroughly. Leave to stand at room temperature for 4–7 days. Stir 2–3 times a day.

Check the taste after 4 days to see how sweet the soda is. The longer it stands, the drier it will get as the sugar is 'eaten up' by the culture. But don't let the soda over-ferment – it should still smell of fresh ginger.

Strain the liquid and bottle into sterilised PET or glass bottles. Don't fill all the way up but leave about 5cm/2in of air in each bottle.

Leave the soda at room temperature for 1–2 days until carbonated. Transfer to the fridge so that the fermentation process is stalled.

CHRISTMAS SODA

My version of what we in Sweden call julmust is a juniper berry soda with Christmas flavours. I normally brew it about a week before Christmas, and then it is carbonated just in time for Christmas Eve.

About 4 litres/7 pints/16 cups
100g/3½oz/¾ cup dried juniper berries, crushed
100g/3½oz/¾ cup raisins
3 prunes
3 dried figs
3 cinnamon sticks (about 4cm/1½in)
100g/3½oz finely chopped fresh root ginger
3 whole mace
10 green cardamom pods
3 cloves
1 star anise
2 pieces dried bitter orange peel
2 tsp citric acid
½ vanilla pod, cut open and seeds scraped out
3.5 litres/6 pints/14 cups water
400g/14oz/2 cups dark muscovado sugar
200ml/7fl oz/scant 1 cup Soda Culture (see page 92)

Mix the juniper berries, dried fruit, spices, bitter almond peel and citric acid in a large pan. Stir in the vanilla pod and seeds and 1 litre/1¾ pints/4⅓ cups of the water and bring to the boil. Simmer for about 20 minutes.

Add the sugar and leave to dissolve in the liquid. Remove from the heat and add the remaining 2.5 litres/4¼ pints/ 10 cups of water. Cover with clingfilm and leave to steep for about 12 hours.

Strain through a fine sieve. Stir in the soda culture and cover with muslin. Leave to stand at room temperature for 3–5 days. Stir 2–3 times a day.

Check the taste after 3 days. The longer it stands, the drier it will be, but don't let it over-ferment – it should still smell fresh. If you hear a fizzing sound when you stir it, it's time to bottle. Strain and bottle into sterilised PET or glass bottles, leaving 5cm/2in air space. Leave the soda at room temperature for 1–2 days until carbonated. Transfer to the fridge and store for up to 4 weeks.

{ **TIP!** If you want to ferment the Christmas Soda using yeast add scant ⅛ tsp instead of soda culture and ferment for 1–2 days in PET bottles just like you do for Fizzy Orange Soda (page 82) or Grapefruit Soda (page 78).

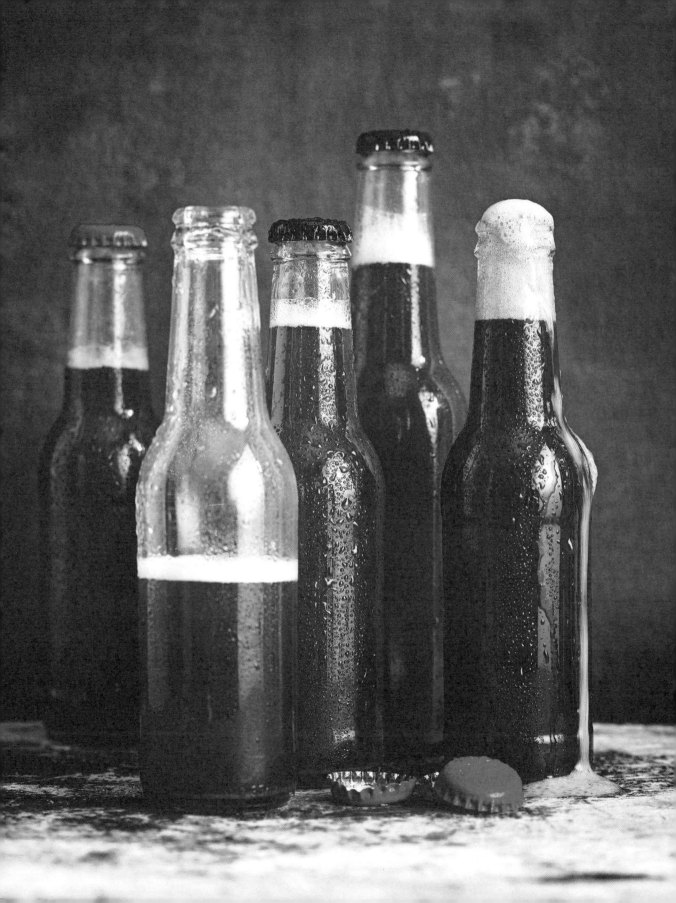

FLOATS
Egg Cream, Iced Coffee
AND BUBBLE TEA

It won't always be the case that you want a dry, sour, bitter and slightly grown-up flavour in your soda or lemonade. Sometimes you crave something sweet and carbonated that's more like a refreshing dessert.

Using syrup or homemade soda as a base, you can easily make a soda float, egg cream or shaved ice. If you want something that resembles milkshake, you can mix up an ice cream soda or the Mexican drink horchata made from rice milk and sweetened with condensed milk. Or why not try a bubble tea with the taste of tea or fruit with tapioca pearls in the bottom of the glass.

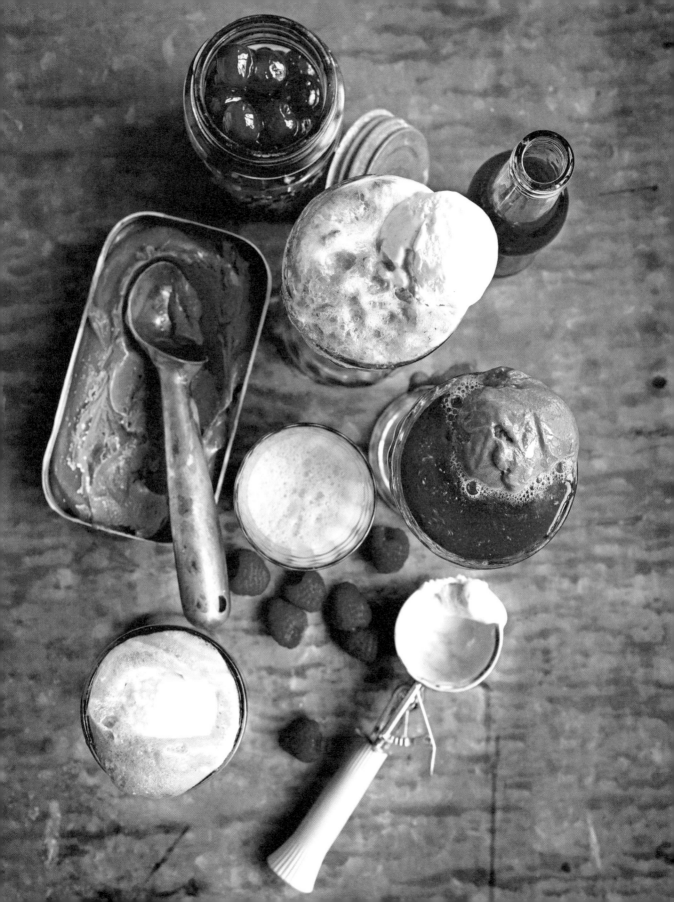

FLOATS

A soda float is a glass of soda, often cola, with a good scoop of ice cream floating on top. When the ice cream gets in contact with the fizzy soda in the glass a bubbly foam that resembles milkshake appears. To make this simple drink a bit more complicated you should, according to the soda experts I talked with when I visited American soda fountains, place the scoop of ice cream towards the side of the glass so that it stays on top and doesn't fall straight down to the bottom of the glass. If you get it right, it will stay there and bubble on top and develop the ultimate soda float foam.

If you make a float from homemade ice cream and homemade cola you get a soda float deluxe. Try to make a float from Salted Caramel Ice Cream (see right) or Raspberry Sorbet (see page 108). Sea Buckthorn Trocadero (page 47) and Salted Caramel Ice Cream together is like a buttery pie dessert in a glass, while Rhubarb, Lime and Lemongrass soda (page 25) with a scoop of Raspberry Sorbet is like a bowl of fresh summer berries with sprightly fizzy bubbles.

ICE CREAM SODA

A kind of milkshake, but with bubbles. Instead of mixing milk and ice cream you mix soda and ice cream.

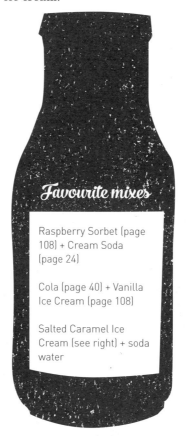

Favourite mixes

Raspberry Sorbet (page 108) + Cream Soda (page 24)

Cola (page 40) + Vanilla Ice Cream (page 108)

Salted Caramel Ice Cream (see right) + soda water

Homemade ice cream
Always cover the freshly made ice cream with a lid or clingfilm before you place it in the freezer, to avoid the ice cream getting icy.

SALTED CARAMEL ICE CREAM

Creamy ice cream with a taste of salted caramel – you will never have tasted anything nicer!

6–8 portions
135g/4¾oz/⅔ cups Demerara sugar
200ml/7fl oz/scant 1 cup whipping cream
300ml/½ pint/1¼ cups semi-skimmed milk
3 tbsp glucose syrup
2 pinches of salt
5 egg yolks

Place a suitable dish or container with a lid in the freezer for the ice cream.

Melt the sugar over a low heat until it turns a golden brown colour and starts to smell like caramel (make sure it doesn't burn). Don't stir!

Add the cream, milk, glucose syrup and salt. Simmer gently until the sugar has dissolved.

Whisk the egg yolks with about 200ml/7fl oz/scant 1 cup of the hot mixture and then whisk in the rest.

Simmer the mixture in a pan until it reaches 82°C/180°F. Leave to cool, then put in the fridge for 2 hours.

Run the ice cream in an ice-cream machine until you get a creamy consistency. Don't let it run in the machine for too long, stop when it's still soft and creamy.

Fill the cold ice cream dish with the ice cream and leave in the freezer for at least 1 hour, or until needed.

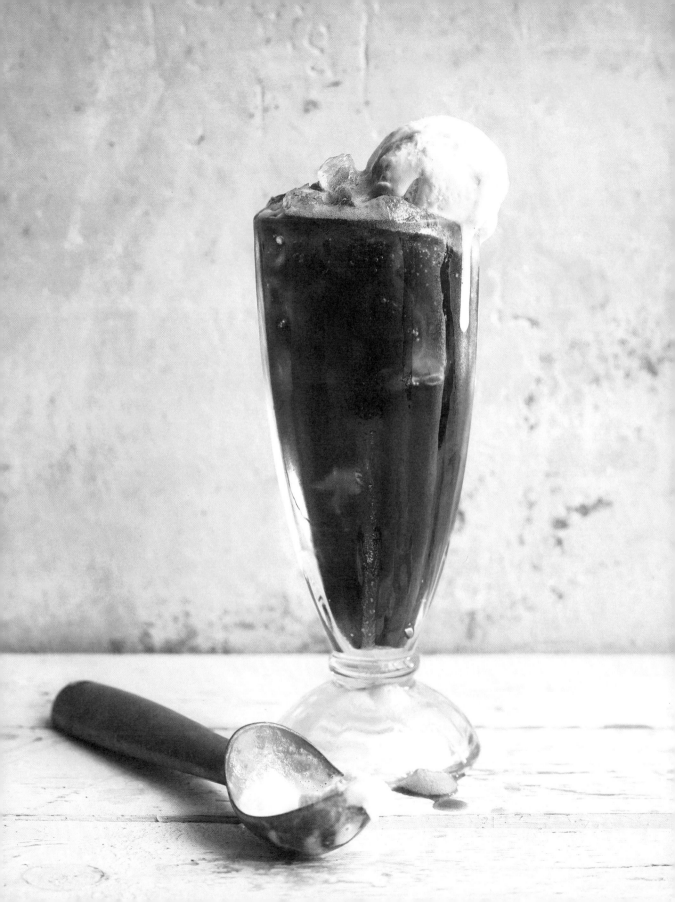

VANILLA ICE CREAM

*The best homemade ice cream –
creamy and full of real vanilla!*

6–8 portions
250g/9oz/generous 1 cup
  whipping cream
250g/9oz/generous 1 cup
  whole milk
1 vanilla pod, cut open and
  seeds scraped out
1 gelatine leaf
6 egg yolks
225g/8oz/1½ cups granulated sugar

Place a suitable dish or
container with a lid in the
freezer for the ice cream.

Heat the cream, milk, vanilla
pod and seeds in a pan. Soak
the gelatine in cold water.
Whisk the egg yolks and sugar
until fluffy. Whisk the hot milk
into the egg mixture, then pour
it back into the pan.

Simmer gently, stirring
constantly, until the mixture
thickens slightly – enough
to lightly coat the back of a
wooden spoon.

Remove from the heat. Gently
squeeze out the water from
the gelatine leaf and whisk it
into the mixture. Take out the
vanilla pod. Leave the creamy
mixture to cool.

Run in an ice-cream machine
for about 40 minutes until
you get a creamy consistency.
Transfer the ice cream to
the cold dish and keep in the
freezer for at least 1 hour or
until needed.

If the ice cream is hard when
you take it out of the freezer
you can leave it for 15 minutes
before serving.

RASPBERRY SORBET

*A dash of yogurt gives a
rounded acidity to this
raspberry sorbet. The
raspberries can be replaced
with other berries, such as
blueberries, strawberries or
red currants, depending on
which kind of soda float you
want to make.*

6–8 portions
225g/8oz/1½ cups granulated
  sugar
3 tbsp glucose syrup
500g/1lb 2oz raspberries
1 gelatine leaf
200ml/7fl oz/scant 1 cup Greek
  yogurt

Melt the sugar and glucose
syrup in a pan until golden
brown. Add the raspberries and
simmer until you have a smooth
raspberry mixture.

Soak the gelatine leaf in cold
water for about 5 minutes.
Blend the raspberry mixture
into a smooth sauce using a
stick blender. Strain the seeds
off through a fine sieve. Mix
the gelatine leaf with the hot
raspberry mixture. Mix with
yogurt and run in an ice-cream
machine until it has a creamy
consistency.

Leave in the freezer for at
least 1 hour, or until needed.

SODA CREAM FIZZ

*Ramos gin fizz is a favourite
cocktail: sour, creamy, fizzy and
with a crown of creamy foam.
This is an alcohol-free version,
but if you feel like something
stronger, splash in a measure
of gin.*

1 glass
2 tbsp simple syrup (see method
  below)
1 egg white
½ tsp orange blossom water
2 tbsp freshly squeezed lemon
  juice (about ½ lemon)
1 tbsp freshly squeezed lime juice
  (about ½ lime)
2 tbsp whipping cream
100ml/3½fl oz/scant ½ cup
  soda water

Mix together a simple syrup
using equal parts water to
sugar (2 tbsp water, 2 tbsp
sugar). Warm in a pan or a
microwave oven, dissolving
the sugar in the liquid. Leave
to cool.

Mix together the egg white,
orange blossom water, simple
syrup, lemon and lime juice
and cream in a cocktail shaker.
Fill with ice and shake until
the shaker has turned ice cold.
Pour into a large glass. Add
soda water so that you get a
proper foam on the surface.
Serve immediately!

SALTY PEANUT BLACK 'N' WHITE COOKIES

Here's a classic New York pairing: egg cream with a black 'n' white cookie. The original resembles a small sponge cake, almost like a Madeleine (but a little drier), that's topped with white and brown icing. This is a black 'n' white cookie mark 2, with peanuts in the batter and chocolate truffle and white topping.

Makes about 30
150g/5½oz/heaped 1 cup salted peanuts
235g/8½oz/scant 2 cups plain flour
1 tsp vanilla sugar
½ tsp baking powder
1 tsp salt
2 eggs
200g/7oz/1 cup granulated sugar
3 tbsp whole milk
125g/4½oz butter, melted

CHOCOLATE ICING
100g/3½oz dark chocolate, finely chopped
4 tbsp whipping cream
25g/1oz butter

WHITE ICING
140g/5oz/1 cup icing sugar
1½ tbsp water
1 tbsp glucose syrup

Preheat the oven to 170°C/325°F and line a baking sheet with baking parchment. Blend the peanuts into a fine powder in a food processor. Mix together the flour, vanilla sugar, baking powder and salt in a bowl.

Whisk together the eggs and sugar using an electric whisk. Add the milk, melted butter and peanuts, then whisk into a smooth batter. Sift the flour mix into the batter and quickly stir until smooth. Leave to rest for about 15 minutes.

Spoon out dollops of the batter onto the prepared baking sheet, about 1 tbsp for each cookie. Leave a 3cm/1¼in gap in between the cookies as they will spread to about 5cm/2in across.

Bake in the centre of the oven for about 12–15 minutes. Leave to cool.

CHOCOLATE ICING: Place the chocolate in a bowl. Bring the cream to the boil and pour over the chocolate. Stir and leave to stand for about 1 minute. Fold in the butter and stir to a smooth paste.

WHITE ICING: Mix the ingredients together in a bowl.

Use a palette knife to spread icing on the flat side of the cookies, one half with white icing and the other half with chocolate icing. Place in the fridge and leave to set. (See photograph on page 110.)

EGG CREAM

Egg cream is a New York classic invented in Brooklyn during the 1920s soda-fountain craze.

Egg cream has nothing to do with eggs or cream but is made from three ingredients: chocolate or vanilla syrup, milk and carbonated water. I like to use a milk with a high fat content for a creamier taste.

In combination with chocolate syrup it's almost like a cross between a milkshake and chocolate milk, but fizzy.

To mix together the perfect egg cream is an art. You must add the different ingredients to the glass in a specific order. First syrup, then milk and finally water. You place a spoon with a long handle in the bottom of the glass and swirl around until you get a white foamy crown on top, otherwise it's a failed egg cream unfortunately.

The professionals say the chocolate syrup should be Fox's U-bet Chocolate Syrup, but it's hard to find outside of New York so I use a homemade syrup. It must be fat-free – so no adding butter or cream to get a more indulgent sauce.

Chocolate and vanilla are the most common egg creams. I like chocolate best. If you want to try vanilla egg cream you can replace chocolate syrup with Cream Soda (page 24) to give a milky toffee-like flavour.

1 glass
CHOCOLATE SYRUP
75g/3oz/scant ½ cup cocoa powder
100g/3½oz/½ cup granulated sugar
100ml/3½fl oz/scant ½ cup water
a small pinch of salt

EGG CREAM
1½ tbsp chocolate syrup
150ml/¼ pint/scant ⅔ cup whole milk
300ml/½ pint/1¼ cups soda water

First make the syrup. Bring all the ingredients to the boil and simmer for about 5 minutes. Leave to cool.

To make the egg cream, follow the instructions above. (See photograph on page 111.)

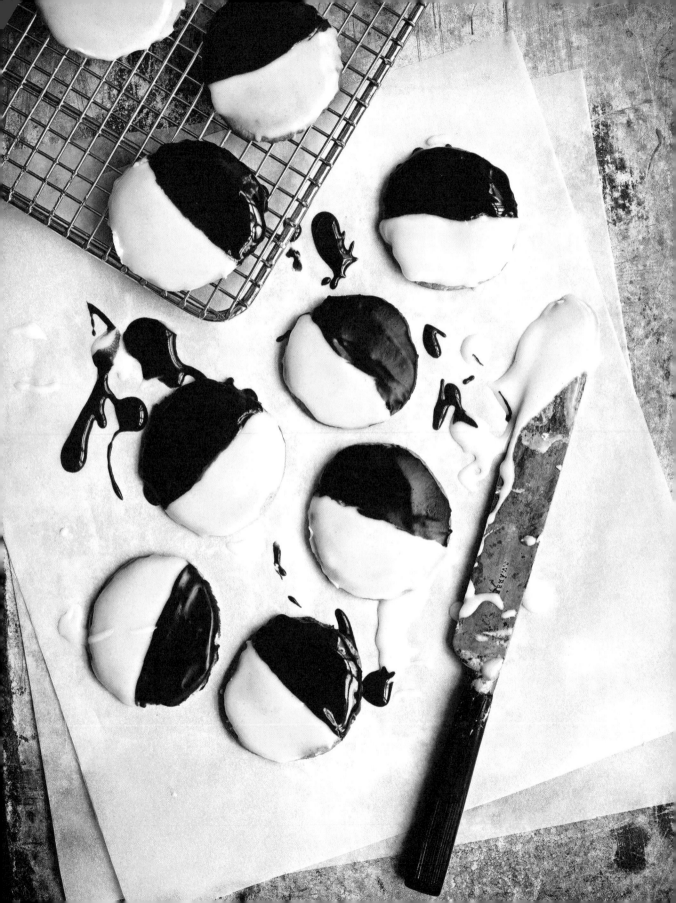

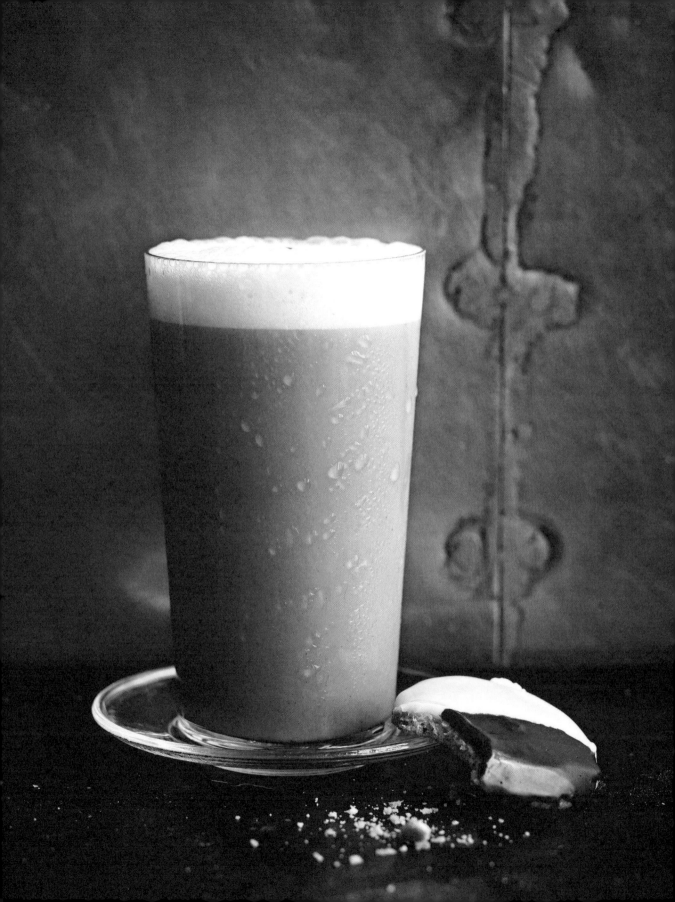

COLD-BREWED
ICED COFFEE

It's all about cold-brewed according to the iced coffee experts, meaning that you don't boil, brew or prepare your coffee using a stove-top coffee maker but instead leave it to gradually steep and then let it slowly strain through a filter. When the coffee is cold-brewed, no bitter compounds or harsh tannins develop that can be a bit dull in an iced coffee. Instead the flowery citrus tones that you can find in coffee come to the fore, and make the drink extra special. It takes about 12 hours to get the finished result – a strong concentrate that is mixed with water and ice, depending on how strong you want it. The concentrate will keep for a long time, up to 2 weeks in the fridge, without losing any flavour or aroma. Iced coffee with milk or without? You decide.

4 cups
100g/3½oz/1 cup coffee beans
450ml/¾ pint/2 cups water

Grind the coffee beans in a coffee grinder or ask for it to be ground at the store. The coffee should be as freshly ground as possible!

Mix the coffee and water together in a jar. Stir. Cover with a lid and leave to stand at room temperature for about 12–24 hours.

Line a sieve with muslin or a large coffee filter. Place the sieve on top of a bowl.

Pour the freshly brewed coffee and leave to drip slowly until all the coffee is gathered in the bowl. Store in the fridge in a jar with a lid.

Mix about half and half of the concentrate and water in a glass filled with ice.

WATERMELON
& LIME SLUSHIE

4 glasses
800g/1lb 12oz watermelon
5 tbsp freshly squeezed lime juice
   (about 1½ limes)
1–2 tbsp clear honey

Peel and slice the melon into cubes. Place in the freezer for at least 3 hours.

Blend the melon and lime juice into a half-frozen slushie using a blender. Add honey to taste and serve immediately.

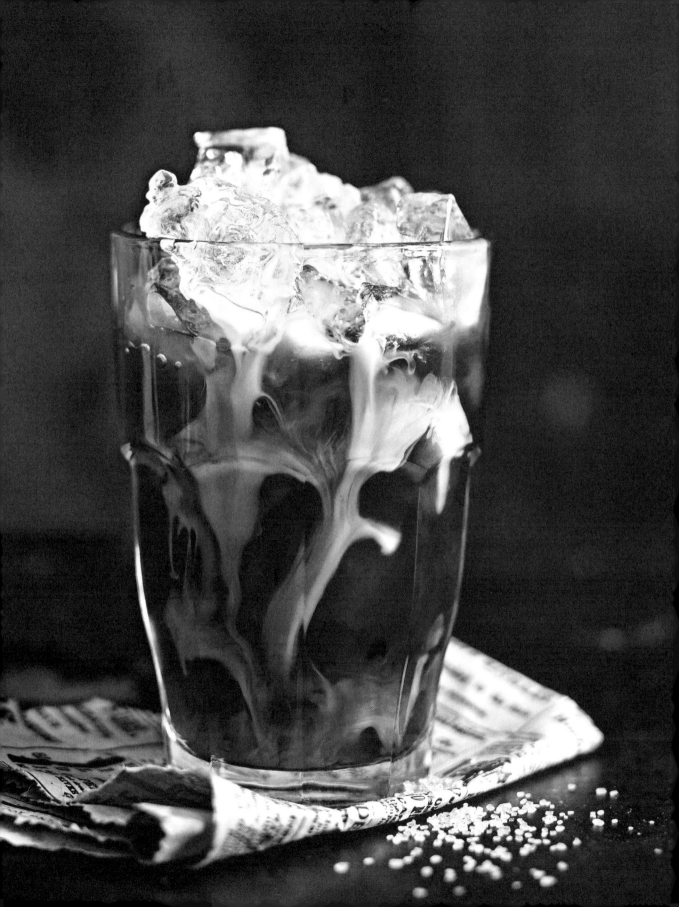

AGUA DE HORCHATA

This Mexican rice and almond milk drink is usually flavoured with cinnamon, but there are also fruity versions like strawberry and cherry. The original is very sweet, almost sickly – my version is a little more refreshing and is only sweetened with condensed milk.

Makes about 6 glasses

130g/4½oz/1 cup blanched
   almonds
100g/3½oz/½ cup white uncooked
   rice, such as basmati
1 cinnamon stick
1 litre/1¾ pints/4⅓ cups water
150ml/¼ pint/scant ⅔ cup
   condensed milk
2 tbsp freshly squeezed lime juice
   (about 1 lime), optional

Toast the almonds in a hot frying pan, they shouldn't get too much colour, just slightly golden brown. Blend the rice into a powder in a food processor. Mix together with almonds and cinnamon stick in a large bowl.

Bring half the water to the boil, then pour it over the rice and almonds. Leave to cool. Cover with clingfilm. Leave to stand for 12 hours in the fridge.

Mix the soaked rice, almonds and cinnamon stick with the rest of the water. Blend into a smooth paste. Strain through a fine sieve into a large jug or bowl.

Mix with the condensed milk. Place in the fridge and serve with ice and a squeeze of lime, if you like.

CHURROS

Churros can be found both in Spain and in South America and are like thin doughnuts. You'll find them in various places: in small cafés in Madrid, on the street in Mexico City or in a churro-making abuela's (granny's) home. Freshly fried and crispy they're dipped into chocolate sauce. Served together with horchata you have the ultimate sweet combo.

Makes about 20

250g/9oz/generous 1 cup water
125g butter
1 tbsp + 200g/7oz/1 cup granulated
   sugar
2 pinches of salt
250g/9oz/2 cups plain flour
2 eggs
1 litre/1¾ pints/4⅓ cups deep-
   frying oil, such as rapeseed
2 tsp ground cinnamon

Heat the water, butter and 1 tbsp sugar in a pan. Add the salt and work in the flour in batches using a wooden spoon.

Remove from the heat and work the dough into a ball that easily comes off the edges of the pan. Leave to rest for 10 minutes so that the dough rises slightly. Add one egg at a time and work into a batter.

Spoon the batter into a piping bag fitted with a small star nozzle. Churros expand in the oil, so if they are too thick they will not be crispy enough.

Heat the oil to 180°C/350°F. Pipe the batter into about 5cm/2in long churros strips straight into the deep-frying oil, about 5 at a time.

Fry until golden brown and crispy, about 4 minutes, flipping them over halfway through.

Take out with a slotted spoon and leave to drain on a piece of kitchen paper.

Mix together the remaining sugar with the cinnamon on a plate. Roll the churros in the sugar while still warm so that the sugar coats them all over. Serve as soon as possible.

Chocolate sauce
Bring 50g/1¾oz butter, 4 tbsp cocoa powder, 100ml/3½fl oz/ scant ½ cup whipping cream, 100g/3½oz/⅔ cup golden syrup and a pinch of salt to the boil in a pan. Leave to simmer for about 10 minutes on a medium heat. Serve warm or cold with churros.

Tip! To get a creamy toffee flavour on your horchata you can let the unopened can of condensed milk simmer in a pan covered with a lid for about 4 hours. The condensed milk will transform into toffee sauce, dulce de leche, which is widely used in Latin America.

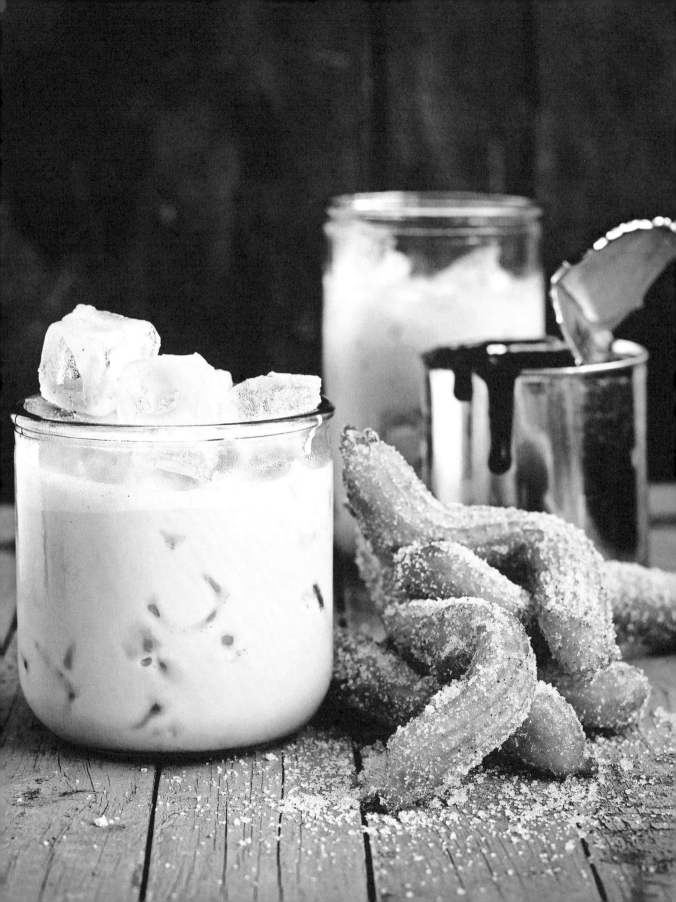

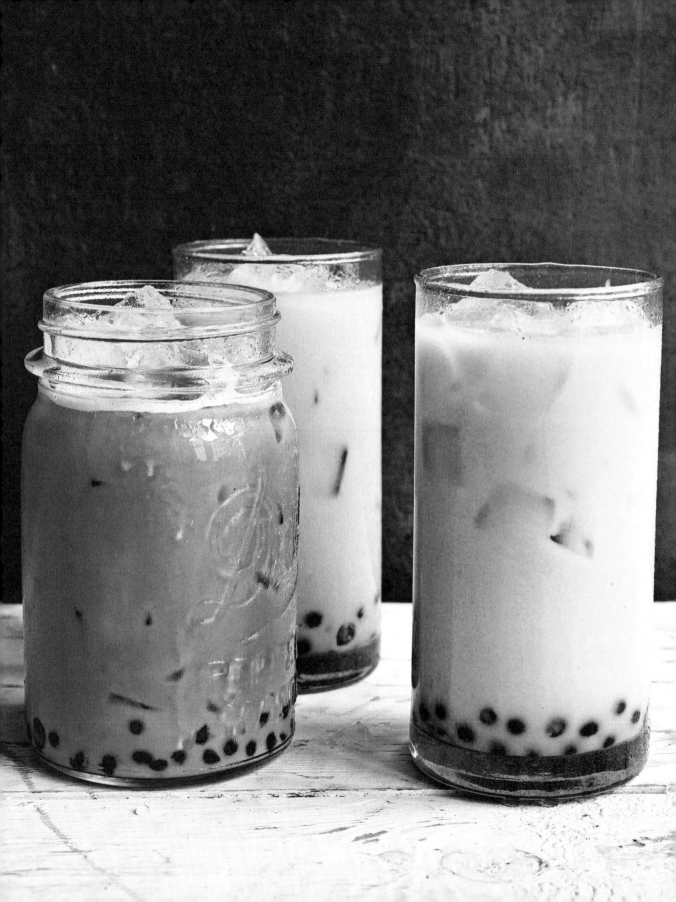

BUBBLE TEA

My version of bubble tea is not quite as sweet as it really should be if you do it according to the rule book. I like it when a drink refreshes instead of makes you even thirstier than you were before drinking it.

The boiled, perfectly chewy black tapioca pearls are nicest freshly boiled, but can also be soaked in a simple syrup and then kept in the fridge for several days. You can find the pearls in Asian food stores or online. Buy the large black pearls; if you use fine tapioca (sago grains) the drink will be too thick.

Bubble tea originates from Taiwan where it was started to be mixed in tea bars in the beginning of the 1980s. The popularity of the drink spread over Asia and to the rest of the world and can now be found bottled. It's tastiest when it's freshly made – the pearls will have the ultimate consistency a few hours after they have been boiled.

BASIC BUBBLE TEA

1 glass
500ml/17fl oz/generous 2 cups water + 150ml/¼ pint/scant ⅔ cup water
4 tbsp black tapioca pearls
225g/8oz/1½ cups granulated sugar
150ml/¼ pint/scant ⅔ cup strong black tea
100ml/3½fl oz/scant ½ cup whole milk or almond milk
1–2 tbsp condensed milk

Bring 500ml/17fl oz/generous 2 cups of the water to the boil in a pan. Add the tapioca pearls and boil for 20 minutes. Turn the heat off and leave to stand, covered with a lid for another 20 minutes.

Boil the 150ml/¼ pint/scant ⅔ cup water together with the sugar to make a simple syrup. Leave to cool.

Drain the tapioca pearls and rinse them in cold water. Place the pearls in the simple syrup and store them in the fridge.

Mix 2 tbsp tapioca pearls with tea, milk and condensed milk in a large glass. Top up with ice.

MATCHA BUBBLE TEA

1 glass
150ml/¼ pint/scant ⅔ cup strong green tea
½ tsp matcha green tea powder
2 tbsp tapioca pearls, cooked according to the basic recipe
100ml/3½fl oz/scant ½ cup whole milk
1–2 tbsp condensed milk

Prepare the tea and mix with the matcha green tea powder. Leave to cool until the drink gets completely cold.

Mix the tapioca pearls with the tea, milk and condensed milk in a large glass. Top up with ice.

BLACK SESAME RICE BUBBLE TEA

1 glass
150ml/¼ pint/scant ⅔ cup strong black tea
2 tbsp black sesame seeds
about 120ml/4fl oz/½ cup condensed milk
2 tbsp tapioca pearls, cooked according to the basic recipe
100ml/3½fl oz/scant ½ cup rice milk

Blend together the tea, sesame seeds and condensed milk using a stick blender. Strain through a fine sieve.

Mix together the tapioca pearls and milk in a large glass. Top up with ice.

FRUITY BUBBLE TEA

1 glass
150ml/¼ pint/scant ⅔ cup strong green tea
1–2 tbsp clear honey
3 tbsp fruit or berry purée, such as raspberry, pomegranate, strawberry, peach, passion fruit, blueberry etc.
100ml/3½fl oz/scant ½ cup whole milk or rice milk
2 tbsp tapioca pearls, cooked according to the basic recipe

Mix together the tea, honey, fruit or berry purée and milk using a blender.

Mix the tapioca pearls with the liquid in a large glass. Top up with ice.

RECIPE INDEX

DRINKS

PLACES TO BUY

Kombucha cultures

Happy Kombucha
www.happykombucha.co.uk

Spices, herbs, roots and bark

Healthy Supplies
www.healthysupplies.co.uk

Just Ingredients
www.justingredients.co.uk

Sous Chef
www.souschef.co.uk

The Spicery
www.thespicery.co.uk

The Spice Shop
www.thespiceshop.co.uk

Yeast, hops and bottles

Cream Supplies
www.creamsupplies.co.uk

The Home Brew Shop
www.the-home-brew-shop.co.uk

Love Brewing
www.lovebrewing.co.uk

THANKS TO EVERYONE WHO HAS HELPED ME WITH MY BOOK!

The absolute best publishing team: publisher Maria Nilsson, editor Elisabeth Fock and publicist Josefin Ekman at Natur & Kultur for enthusiastic test cooking, fun collaboration and because you always publish cookery books that you want to read!

Katy Kimbell for pretty design and illustration!

Wolfgang Kleinschmidt for equally fantastic photography and because it's always fun to work with you!

Karin Lundin because you do that little extra with the images!

My Robin who's coped with drinking successful and unsuccessful soda during the whole of 2013!

My family and my friends for support, inspiration, cheering and testing of all things carbonated and deep-fried!